American Heart
Association.
Fighting Heart Disease and Stroke

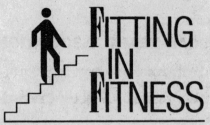

FITTING IN FITNESS

Also by the
AMERICAN HEART ASSOCIATION

American Heart Association Cookbook, 5th Edition

American Heart Association Low-Fat, Low-Cholesterol Cookbook

American Heart Association Low-Salt Cookbook

American Heart Association Quick and Easy Cookbook

American Heart Association Around the World Cookbook

American Heart Association Kids' Cookbook

American Heart Association Guide to Heart Attack

American Heart Association Family Guide to Stroke

American Heart Association 6 Weeks to Get Out the Fat

American Heart Association Brand Name Fat and Cholesterol Counter

With the American Cancer Society Living Well, Staying Well

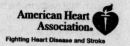

American Heart
Association®

Fighting Heart Disease and Stroke

FITTING IN FITNESS

Hundreds of
Simple Ways to
Put More
Physical Activity
into Your Life

Clarkson Potter/Publishers
New York

Your contribution to the American Heart Association supports research that helps make publications like this possible. For more information, call 1-800-AHA-USA1 (1-800-242-8721) or contact us online at http://www.amhrt.org.

Published by Clarkson Potter/Publishers, New York, New York. Member of the Crown Publishing Group.

Random House Inc. New York, Toronto, London, Sydney, Auckland
www.randomhouse.com

CLARKSON N. POTTER is a trademark and POTTER and colophon are registered trademarks of Random House, Inc.

Originally published by Times Books in 1997.

Printed in the United States of America

Book design by Leon Bolognese & Associates, Inc.

Library of Congress Cataloging-in-Publication Data
American Heart Association fitting in fitness: hundreds of simple ways to put more physical activity into your life.
   1. Exercise.   2. Physical fitness.   I. American Heart Association
RA781.A58   1997
613.7'1—dc21   96-49730

ISBN 0-8129-2911-X

24 23 22 21 20 19 18 17 16

No book, including this one, can ever replace the services of a physician. It's a good idea to check with your doctor before starting this or any other health program. Although we cannot guarantee any results, we hope this book will help you both attain your goals for better health and work more effectively with your doctor.

FOREWORD

The facts are clear. As a nation, we're out of shape. We simply do not get enough physical activity. Sadly, most people's workdays and leisure time are spent sitting—working at computers, in meetings, commuting, or watching television. In fact, the recent *Surgeon General's Report on Physical Activity and Health* said that more than 60 percent of American adults are not regularly physically active and at least 25 percent are not active at all.

Being inactive and unfit has a negative effect on your health. Many studies show that a sedentary lifestyle is associated with an increased risk for heart disease, obesity, high blood pressure, colon cancer, diabetes, and osteoporosis. Low fitness also affects your quality of life. For example, regular physical activity seems to enhance psychological well-being and physical functioning, especially in your later years.

The evidence keeps growing. Recent research from our center has confirmed that moderately fit people have a considerably lower risk of dying prematurely than people with a low fitness level. The study also showed this shocker: Poor physical fitness is as important a predictor of premature death as cigarette smoking, high blood pressure, and high blood cholesterol.

The good news is that most people can easily achieve a healthful fitness level. The *Surgeon General's Report* recommends that both children and adults include a minimum of thirty minutes of moderate-level physical activity (such as brisk walking) on most, preferably all, days.

The best news is that you don't have to get your thirty minutes all at once. And you don't have to do it in a gym.

That's how this book can help you. It gives you hundreds of creative ways to fit in physical activity throughout your day. Seemingly minor strategies such as taking the stairs instead of the elevator and parking farther away from your destination can add up over time to better fitness and health if you do them regularly. Once you get used to fitting in fitness in your daily routine, you may want to do even more. Studies show that doing vigorous or moderate activities for longer durations will yield even higher levels of fitness and greater health benefits.

No single solution can solve all the health problems in this country. I'm convinced, however, that if Americans would get up off their chairs and start moving as part of their normal, everyday routine, we would make great strides toward increasing the longevity and quality of life for people of all ages.

— Steven N. Blair, P.E.D., director of research,
   Cooper Institute for Aerobics Research,
   Dallas, Texas; senior scientific editor,
   *Surgeon General's Report on Physical
   Activity and Health*

ACKNOWLEDGMENTS

When we started this book, the most exercise some of us got in our daily lives was turning on the computer. Oh, don't get us wrong. We walked or bicycled when we could. But when we couldn't, we often just sat.

Now each of us has learned at least a dozen new ways to fit in fitness every day, rain or shine. We've found how easy it is to add thirty minutes of activity to an average workday. And the best news is this: That's all it takes to get the health benefits of regular exercise!

Now it's *your* turn.

We packed this book with everything we could think of to keep you moving—at the office, on the road, while shopping, at home, with kids. You'll find hundreds of ways to fit fitness into your everyday life—and heart health into your future.

Our exercise experts, Ruth Ann Carpenter, M.S., R.D., and DeeDee McCabe, B.S., researched or devised all the activities in this book. They're staff members of the Cooper Institute for Aerobics Research, a nonprofit preventive medicine research and education center in Dallas, Texas. Ruth Ann already stays fit by bicycling. Even she learned some new fitness tricks by working on this guide. On a recent eleven-hour plane ride to Germany, she took advantage of the time by doing isometric exercises. And even though DeeDee routinely runs for exercise, she has recently started walking and doing squats and stretches when she's on the phone at home.

American Heart Association managing editor Jane Anneken Ruehl corralled this team of experts, writers, and editors and coordinated the development process from concept to completed book. An avid tennis player, she now tries to arrive early for meetings so she can walk around the block a couple of times before they begin.

Janice Roth Moss, AHA editor and self-proclaimed couch potato, painstakingly copyedited every word of this book. She used to combine chores to save time but has become an advocate of "planned inefficiencies." She thinks the time is well spent because she's now improving her fitness. And writer Pat Harmon Naegele, who smoothed out and punched up the words of the experts, now regularly takes the stairs instead of the elevator.

Finally, AHA science consultant Terry Bazzarre, Ph.D., FACSM, pored over this book, checking the accuracy of every fact and fitness tip. Terry already walks his dogs about two miles a day. He's been traveling a lot lately and now incorporates some of the fitness-on-the-road tips into his travel routine.

As you can see, this book has changed our lives. In big ways and little ways. We hope it all adds up to heart health. We also hope you'll join us. We're proof positive that you can't read this book without walking away with new fitness ideas and a new attitude. Good luck!

CONTENTS

INTRODUCTION

You know you should be more physically active. You even *want* to be. But where will you find the time? And just how active do you have to be? *Fitting in Fitness* will help you find the answers.

♡ *The Couch Potato Epidemic*

We understand your dilemma. For an astounding number of us, walking to the sofa and turning on the TV is the most physical activity we get in a day. Thanks to the ever-ready car, elevators, escalators, and sedentary jobs, we hardly have to move at all. And it's costing us plenty in heart disease and stroke, often as early as in midlife. At the American Heart Association, we know that physical inactivity is a major risk factor for heart attack and stroke. In fact, each year about 250,000 deaths in the United States are attributed to the lack of regular physical activity.

If you're a couch potato, the good news is that you can help reduce your risk of heart disease simply by filling your day with short bursts of physical activity. You can get the fitness and health benefits you need without a formal, structured exercise program. You're holding the answer in your hands right now. This *Fitting in Fitness* handbook is designed to help you get off the sofa and get moving with minimum hassle and maximum results. There's more good news. You don't have to be a jock. You don't have to run a marathon. You just have to *move*.

♡ Sneaking Up on Fitness

On the following pages, you'll learn how walking the dog, taking out the garbage, shopping, traveling, cleaning house, and gardening can actually improve your overall fitness and give you the health benefits of regular exercise.

Although these activities *do* get you up and moving, they don't seem at all like "exercise." These and hundreds of other simple, everyday activities will help you burn calories and help improve your overall fitness.

♡ Research to the Rescue

Interestingly, this book wouldn't have been possible a short time ago. Until then, medical scientists and physiologists thought that only regular, sustained, vigorous activity provided cardiovascular health benefits. But recent research has revealed an amazing fact: People who are moderately active on a regular basis can reap some of the health benefits of more vigorous levels of physical activity. Some recent studies have shown that just being more active can help us feel better and look better, as well as reduce our risk of heart disease. That's why the AHA developed this book. And the more physically active you are, the more benefits you receive.

Best of all, the new research shows that you don't have to do all your physical activity at one time. Instead of taking one thirty-minute walk a day, you can get health benefits even if you split your walk into several shorter segments. If you are just beginning, your goal is to *accumulate* thirty minutes or more of moderate activity each day. If you've been inactive, start off slowly and build your pace over a period of weeks. Regardless of your fitness level, try to accumulate a total of thirty minutes of moderate activity each day, most days of the week. Walking breaks and activities such as gardening and house-cleaning are good ways to do this. For cardiovascular fitness, aim for a total of thirty to sixty minutes of vigorous physical activity each day, three to four days per week.

Aim for segments of at least ten minutes of activity. That's not always practical, though, and any activity is better than none.

It's true that playing sports for thirty minutes can also give you the health benefits you need, but that's not what this book is all about. We're offering a "lifestyle approach" to physical activity. We're suggesting that you can simply "fit in fitness" with your current lifestyle. How? By adding short segments of physical activity to your everyday routine. This approach works if you're totally sedentary now and want to get up and get moving. It also works if you're somewhat active and want to supplement your regular exercise routine.

On these pages, you'll find ways to fit in fitness at home, at work, on the road, with your kids, and when you least expect to be able to. We'll show you hundreds of ways to pack your day with physical activity—and your life with fitness and health.

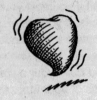

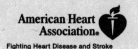

American Heart
Association®

Fighting Heart Disease and Stroke

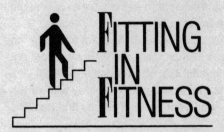

FITTING IN FITNESS

WHAT IS FITNESS?

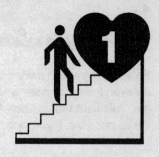

"It is better to wear out one's shoes than one's sheets."
—Genoese proverb

When you think about physical fitness, what comes to mind? Muscular men and women posing for bodybuilding contests? Well, they are strong and look fit, but strong muscles are only one part of total fitness. Those bodybuilders may not be flexible enough to reach an item on a high shelf.

Do you think of fitness as simply the opposite of fatness (if you're slender like a model, you're fit)? Super-sleek fashion models may not be able to lift their own suitcases.

In addition to strength, total fitness includes endurance and flexibility. Total fitness means being able to touch your toes and climb a couple of flights of stairs without gasping for breath.

♡ Energy for Everyday Life

Basically, fitness is having the energy and strength to do everything you need and want to do in your daily life. You want that not only for today but for as late in life as possible. If you're fit, you can:

○ Keep up with today's fast-paced society

○ Carry an armload of groceries into the house

○ Actively play with your children or grandchildren

○ Fully enjoy your retirement years

○ Continue to take care of yourself as you grow older

○ Avoid nursing-home care as long as possible

During childhood and adolescence, you may have gradually developed a fitness level through active play, games, and sports. As you age, you may slowly begin to lose some of this fitness if you are inactive. People who stay active throughout their lifespan can delay the loss of strength, flexibility, and endurance that's associated with aging.

D ID YOU KNOW . . .

Of Americans who consider themselves frequent exercisers, 76 percent are over age thirty-five.

♡ *So, Are Fat and Flab Inevitable?*

Although no magic pill or potion will stop you from losing some fitness as you age, you *can* slow the process dramatically. In some cases, you might even reverse it! How? With regular physical activity.

That doesn't mean you have to be a marathon runner, a basketball superstar, or a decathlon champion. For most people, physical activity simply means moving. And it doesn't really matter what you do—digging in your garden, playing outside with your kids, vacuuming, cleaning out the attic. What counts is just getting out and doing *something*.

In this book, we'll show you some simple ways to put more of this fitness-enhancing movement into your life. You'll find lots of things you can do anytime, anywhere to add to your overall physical fitness.

Whether you're twenty or sixty, physical activity is at least as important to your health as not smoking cigarettes and eating low-fat foods. In fact, some studies have shown that physically inactive people have the same risk of heart disease as people who smoke *two packs of cigarettes a day.* The bottom line? If you want to be healthy, get *moving*!

♡ *But Wait, There's MORE!*

Physical activity brings you a lot more than fitness. If it helps keep you healthy, it means a wonderful, vibrant quality of life—for a lifetime.

Americans spend billions of dollars a year on medical treatments to cure lifestyle-related diseases that rob them of their vitality. Unsuspecting, often desperate consumers spend billions more on quack treatments. Sadly, if those people had quit (or never started) smoking, cut down on high-fat foods, and been physically active, they might have prevented their illnesses.

Of course, exercise is not a magic cure. However, it *is* a critical part of staying healthy. Studies have shown that regular physical activity can help:

○ Reduce your risk of heart disease

○ Improve blood circulation

○ Lower your risk of developing diabetes

○ Manage your weight

○ Slow the natural loss of bone mass

○ Reduce your risk of colon cancer

○ Strengthen your muscles, bones, and joints

○ Reduce high blood pressure

○ Relieve tension and anxiety

○ Improve your energy level

○ Boost your self-confidence and self-esteem

○ Improve older adults' ability to move about without falling

Studies also have shown that people at the highest fitness levels are far less likely to die prematurely *for any reason* (such as heart disease, cancer, even accidents) than those at the lowest fitness levels. Researchers have learned that physically active people get immediate benefits from the activity. The more activity, the more these benefits build up. The people in the most danger lead sedentary lives. The message of this new research is clear: It doesn't matter how physically active you are, it matters that you at least do *something*.

Even when you realize how critical regular physical activity is, you may have a hard time making yourself begin. Millions of people wake up every morning with excuses for not moving off dead center. Are you one of them?

♡ *Yes! So What's Holding Me Back?*

If you can't seem to get moving, don't feel alone. In the United States, physical inactivity is at epidemic proportions. More than 60 percent of Americans are not regularly physically active. At least 25 percent are totally sedentary. So what holds these people back? Here are the reasons commonly given for not exercising. Circle the ones that you've used.

"I Don't Have Time"

This is the number one reason Americans give for not being active. If you have this problem, we have some

good news. You don't have to spend hours at a gym
every day to get health benefits from physical activity.
If you're sedentary, all you need is thirty minutes or
more of moderate physical activity on most days. The
news gets even better. You don't have to do the
thirty minutes all at once. You can spread your
activity throughout the day!

"I Can't Afford It"

Adding physical activity to your life doesn't need to
mean joining an exclusive club or buying expensive
equipment. The truth is, you'll find lots of ways to be
physically active. And most of them cost very little or
nothing. All it takes is a little creativity. Keep reading.
By the end of this book, you'll know dozens of ways
to add physical activity to your daily life—without
even touching your wallet.

"I Don't Like to Exercise"

Basic training in the military, high-pressure health
clubs, injuries from improper equipment or programs,
and being picked last for games in gym class are all
reasons people give for hating exercise. Who can
blame them?

Fortunately, you don't have to "go for the burn" or
be a jock to benefit from activity. The key is to find
things you like to do. Think back to your childhood.
Perhaps you enjoyed bike riding, jumping rope, or
swimming. These are all things you can do today. Did
you know that gardening counts as physical activity?
Vigorous weeding, raking, and digging are up there

with playing touch football or volleyball. And remember, you don't have to stick to just one thing! Try a variety of physical activities so that you don't get bored.

"I'm Too Old"

You may think that your forty-something, fifty-something, sixty-something, or seventy-something body can't possibly start being physically active *now*. But research shows otherwise. Studies of people in their *eighties* show that they can reduce the risk of falling and can improve their ability to perform daily activities with a moderate strength-building program. In fact, the older you are, the more important it is to be active if you want to stay vigorous and keep your same lifestyle. Age by itself is simply not a factor. People of any age can do all the activities described in this book.

"I'm Too Tired to Exercise"

This is really the best argument *for* exercise. Being active can actually *boost* your energy! Physically active people report being more energetic, being stronger, and having more stamina. That's because activity makes your heart beat stronger so it pumps blood more efficiently. Your brain, heart, and muscles get more oxygen, so they work better, too. Fitness gives you energy and strength for life.

"I Could Get Hurt"

Regular physical activity doesn't hurt most healthy adults if they *gradually* work up to the amount of activity they want to maintain. Most often, injuries happen when people do too much too soon. The activities you'll find in this book are safe for just about anyone. Simply take the "Do I Need a Medical Okay?" quiz on page 33 before adding more physical activity to your life.

"I'm Too Fat"

Recent research shows that even if you're over-weight, you can be physically fit. In fact, some research suggests that overweight people who are physically fit are less likely to die prematurely than people of normal weight who are unfit! An extra benefit is that if you want to lose weight, regular physical activity and healthful food choices are the best way to help lose it and keep it off.

"None of My Friends Exercise"

It's hard to do things that are different from what your friends and family do. In addition, you'll probably need the support of family and friends to stay active for a lifetime. It's likely they'd also benefit from becoming more active, so urge them to join you. Share the ideas in this book, or get them a copy. By including friends and loved ones in your physical activities, you're doing more than helping yourself.

"I Don't Like to Sweat"

You don't have to sweat to be physically active. You can walk to a neighbor's house, climb two flights of stairs, do stretching activities on a plane, or bicycle to the corner store without changing clothes or perspiring. Yet these all qualify as physical activity.

You may have another reason for not being active. Still, it's easy to see that the rewards of fitness make these reasons look pretty puny. You can be strong, stay healthy, look good, and feel better just by using the stairs at work, walking the dog every evening, and gardening on the weekend. What a trade-off!

♡ *Making the Most of Fitness*

Not all physical activities give you the same benefits. Some strengthen your heart, lungs, and blood vessels. Some help strengthen your bones and muscles. Others help your joints and muscles stay limber. For optimum health, you need a balance of all types of physical activity. The lists below shows how different types of activity help different parts of your body.

To improve your . . .

- ♦ Heart and lungs
- ♦ Muscular strength and endurance
- ♦ Flexibility

You need to . . .

- ♦ Do aerobic activities
- ♦ Do strength-building activities
- ♦ Do stretching activities

♡ The Big Three—Aerobic Capacity, Strength, and Flexibility

For true fitness, you need aerobic, strength-building, *and* flexibility activities. In this book, we offer a balanced, realistic approach to improving your all-around good health by increasing all three kinds of physical activity in your daily life. So, let's get going!

Aerobic Activities

Perhaps your fitness goal is to walk up three flights of stairs without breathing heavily. Or go biking in the country. Or walk in the AHA's annual American Heart Walk. These activities require endurance, and aerobic activities build endurance.

Aerobic means "oxygen." Aerobic activities help you work your heart and lungs, improving your ability to take in oxygen. The better your body uses oxygen, the more active you can be without tiring.

It works like this. The more physically active you are, the more oxygen your body needs to do the activities. You breathe faster and your heart beats faster to deliver more oxygen to the working muscles. Ultimately, the increased workload on your heart makes it stronger and more efficient. Then you can do more without tiring.

In general, aerobic activities use the large muscles in your legs, arms, and back steadily and rhythmically. Aerobic activities include

- ◆ Walking
- ◆ Digging vigorously
- ◆ Bicycling
- ◆ Dancing
- ◆ Raking leaves
- ◆ Hiking
- ◆ Vacuuming quickly
- ◆ Climbing stairs
- ◆ Mopping
- ◆ Skating
- ◆ Swimming
- ◆ Jogging

You can do most of these aerobic activities at different intensity levels. Take walking, for example. You can stroll along at a very leisurely pace—say, twenty minutes per mile. You can pick up the pace and walk at about fifteen to sixteen minutes per mile. You can also walk at a very vigorous pace, less than fifteen minutes per mile. Some people can *walk* faster than others can jog!

Does it matter how intensely you do any given activity? The answer is yes and no. Yes, because you can get greater health benefits by doing more-vigorous activity. No, because if you're inactive now, *any* aerobic activity—regardless of intensity—is better than nothing!

If you've been sedentary, it's not a good idea to begin by doing vigorous activities. Ever tried to go out and run 3 miles after being sedentary for years? All you got was sore muscles, sore knees, and a sore attitude about physical activity!

What counts, then, is the *total amount* of aerobic activity that you do. For some health benefits, begin with a moderate amount of various activities. The chart on page 14 shows that you can get benefits in two ways. You can do either longer sessions of moderately intense activities (such as brisk walking) or shorter sessions of more-vigorous activities (such as running).

What It Takes to Reap Health Benefits

Washing and waxing a car for 45 to 60 minutes

Washing windows or mopping for 45 to
   60 minutes

Playing volleyball for 45 minutes

Playing touch football for 30 to 45 minutes

Gardening for 30 to 45 minutes

Wheeling yourself in a wheelchair for
   30 to 45 minutes

Walking 1³/₄ miles in 35 minutes
   (20 min/mile)

Shooting baskets for 30 minutes

Bicycling 5 miles in 30 minutes

Dancing fast (social dancing) for 30 minutes

Pushing a baby in a stroller 1¹/₂ miles in
   30 minutes

Raking leaves for 30 minutes

Walking 2 miles in 30 minutes (15 min/mile)

Doing water aerobics for 30 minutes

Swimming laps for 20 minutes

Playing wheelchair basketball for 20 minutes

Playing basketball for 15 to 20 minutes

Bicycling 4 miles in 15 minutes

Jumping rope for 15 minutes

Running 1¹/₂ miles in 15 minutes
   (10 min/mile)

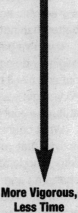

**Less
Vigorous,
More Time**

**More Vigorous,
Less Time**

Getting the physical activity you need is easy. Just pick some things you like to do. If you can't do all your activity at one time, do several shorter sessions. In fact, one study showed that the participants who walked several times a day were better able to sustain a walking program than another group of participants who did the same amount of walking only once a day.

Strength-Building Activities

You may not think of yourself as a weightlifter, but you are. Every time you pick up a child, carry an armload of groceries, or push a heavy box, you're exerting a significant force by a muscle or a muscle group. The stronger your muscles, the more force you can exert.

As you get older, you tend to lose muscle strength. You may have noticed that grandparents have a harder time picking up small children than the parents do. Diminished muscle strength can limit the ability of very old people to do the basic activities of daily living, such as bathing, dressing, and cooking. Physical inactivity is a major factor in this loss of muscle strength. In essence, if you don't use it, you lose it.

Muscular strength can help prevent injuries and reduce lower back pain. It can also help improve your posture and your overall ability in sports, such as golf and tennis. Strong muscles will help you do more vigorous physical activities (shoveling snow, chopping wood, and hiking up a mountain) with less fatigue. Strength training helps preserve lean body mass, which becomes more important as you get older.

So how do you keep your muscles strong? By challenging them with a resistance or a load. In time, your muscles adapt to the challenge by getting stronger. An easy and convenient way to build strength is with calisthenics, such as sit-ups, push-ups, leg lifts, and squats. In calisthenics, you use your body weight as the resistance on certain muscle groups.

Of course, you can use hand weights and weight machines to build strength. If you'd rather not buy this equipment, no problem. You can get the same results from lifting jugs of water. It's not *what* you lift, it's the weight that counts. We'll show you a host of ordinary items around the house and at work that you can use to help improve your muscular strength.

Stretching Activities

Stretching comes naturally. After sitting for hours at a computer or on a plane, have you ever found yourself stretching your back or moving your head from side to side to stretch your neck muscles? It feels so good!

Stretching is great for relieving tension, but that's just one of its many benefits. Stretching before and after exercise helps keep your muscles from tightening up. It also promotes flexibility by allowing your muscles and joints to extend and contract more fully. Staying flexible is especially important as we age, because muscles and joints tend to become less limber. That can lead to stiffness, reduced movement, and increased risk of injury.

Stretching activities are easy to do. Most require

no equipment, and you can do them in less than two minutes. Remember to stretch only until you begin to feel a *slight* pull. (If you feel discomfort, you're stretching too much. You should gradually move through a range of motion until you feel some gentle tension.) Then hold that position for up to thirty seconds. Please, *don't* bounce! Relax, then stretch again. You'll probably find you can stretch a little bit further the second time. This indicates you've improved your muscle's flexibility.

♡ Fitting in Fitness

When it comes to getting more exercise, many people take the "planned exercise" approach. That is, they work out at a moderate or vigorous intensity for at least thirty minutes, with warm-up and cool-down periods, at least three times a week. Sometimes they join a health club, rec center, or exercise class. Some people are very successful at keeping up this amount of activity and can maintain a high level of fitness. Many others, though, fall into the "two weeks on, four months off" school of exercise.

A second method is a bit mellower but no less effective. We call it the lifestyle approach. It's based on the understanding that *some* physical activity is better than *no* physical activity. You can fit physical activity into your day when it's convenient. What matters is the total activity time that you can accumulate in a day.

Surprisingly, although the programmed method may net results faster, it actually requires more time than the lifestyle method. Take a look at the comparison in the table below.

Time Needed to Do a 30-Minute "Workout"

Programmed Activity		Lifestyle Activity	
Activity	*Time (minutes)*	*Activity*	*Time (minutes)*
Drive to gym	5	Walk before work	10
Change clothes	5	Walk at lunch	10
Warm up	5	Walk to and from a	
Take aerobics class	30	neighbor's house	10
Cool down	5		
Change clothes and shower	20		
Drive home	5		
Total Time	**75**	**Total Time**	**30**

The planned exercise approach works well if you are pretty fit and have time to exercise on a regular basis. If, however, you're like most Americans, you don't get enough exercise and you're crunched for time. The lifestyle approach is a great place to start. Most lifestyle physical activities can be done anytime, anywhere, by just about anyone. Most important, in today's time-starved society, you can easily fit this approach into your everyday lifestyle. Later, you may want to add some programmed activity. In fact, the people who are most successful at staying active combine programmed activity with lifestyle activity.

♡ *You Call This Progress?*

Over the decades, our culture and the growth of technology have encouraged us to live sedentary lives. In the name of "progress," we have eliminated many opportunities for physical activities.

Take a look at our work history, for example. In the past, many people used to work hard every day in the fields. As technology improved, they began walking to work at factories in the cities. With the dawn of mass transportation, a walk to the bus stop at the end of the street was all that was needed. Then, with the internal combustion engine, personal transportation, the car, came along. Soon we simply walked to the garage, drove to work, and tried to park as close to the building as possible. We barely had to walk at all. Today, with the advent of the computer and telecommuting, many of us simply roll out of bed, walk to the other side of the house, and start working. What progress! No working hard in the fields, no walking, hardly moving all day except for our fingers whispering rhythmically on the computer keyboard.

Over the years, we've also created tools to save us from hard physical labor. For example, people used to cut the lawn with hand-held sickles. Then the sickle was put on a drum with wheels so they could push the blades across the lawn. Next, the mower was motorized so the blades could spin around and cut the grass. But that still required pushing, so someone attached a belt from the motor to the wheels. Now all we have to do is walk behind the self-propelled wonder. Or we can sit on a riding mower while the machine does all the work. Many of us just hand the riding mower to a neighbor's kid who does the lawn for us!

♡ *Too Smart for Our Own Good?*

These and other technological improvements have saved us time and energy. On the other hand, they have contributed to major health risks caused by physical inactivity. Giving up all the modern amenities isn't the answer, though. The answer is to find ways to replace that much-needed physical activity by thinking differently, being creative, and being adventurous.

♡ *Think Differently*

Before you can improve your body and your health, you need to change your mind. Specifically, you need to change your thinking. We've been trained to think that efficiency is doing more in less time. For example, you may think that talking with your neighbor on the phone is the most "efficient" way to communicate with her. You could sit in your kitchen and talk to her for ten minutes. But wouldn't you both get more benefit if you agreed to meet for a walk and talked then? That way you could accomplish two things instead of just one.

Today, we need to think in terms of "planned inefficiency." Instead of regarding physical activities as time robbers, find ways to fit them into things you already do. They may seem inefficient at first, but try to view these planned inefficiencies as chances to be more active. Take a look at these examples of planned inefficiencies:

- Walking into the bank instead of using the drive-up window
- Walking around the outside aisles at the grocery store at least once before starting your shopping
- Taking the stairs instead of the elevator or escalator
- Parking as far from the door as you can
- Walking to get lunch instead of having it delivered
- Taking only part of the clean laundry upstairs at one time and making more trips
- Getting off the bus a few stops before your destination and walking the rest of the way
- Walking to the airport gate instead of taking a shuttle

CONVENIENCE ISN'T EVERYTHING

Consider avoiding some of the modern technology that makes life more convenient. A small step back to the past can be a step forward for your health.

- Use a push lawn mower or push a self-propelled lawn mower.
- Use manual lawn trimmers and edgers.
- Get on your hands and knees and scrub your floors.
- Wash your car instead of going through a car wash.

♡ Be Creatively Active

Look at how you do things now, and then plan creative ways to build in physical activity. You might spark the creative process by looking for ways to turn "onefers" into "twofers." A onefer is a task or habit you're already doing. To make a onefer a twofer, you simply pair a physical activity with your onefer. We mentioned one example in "Think Differently" on page 20. Here are some others:

Onefers	Twofers
Spending time watching TV with child	Spending time walking with child
Vacuuming	Doing lunges as you vacuum (see page 146)
Talking on the phone	Doing strength-building activities (upper-arm curls, side arm raises, leg lifts, leg kicks) while talking
Standing by the photocopy machine while waiting for your copies	Using the copy machine or a nearby wall so you can do standing push-ups while waiting
Sitting in a traffic jam	Doing stretching activities for your neck and shoulders (you can probably use the tension release!)
Sitting in a meeting with a colleague	Conducting your meeting as you both go for a walk
Driving to the store for a few missing ingredients	Bicycling to the store

A good way to find onefers that you can turn into twofers is to keep a diary of your daily activities for a week or two. Here's how:

1. Get a notepad or notebook.

2. Make two columns on several pages. Write "Onefers" at the top of the left column. Put "Twofers" at the top of the right column.

3. Carry the notepad with you everywhere you go for at least a week (including the weekends).

4. In the Onefers column, as you do different things at home and at work, write them all down. Look at the example below.

Onefers	Twofers
Let the dog out	
Carpool kids to school	
Get coffee	
Talk on phone	
Sit at computer	
Go to lunch	
Sit at child's soccer practice	
Mow yard	

At the end of a week or two, fill in the right columns with a physical activity that you can add to each of your onefer daily activities.

Here's where your creative juices kick in. Don't worry if you can't come up with a twofer for every onefer. Some daily tasks simply don't lend themselves to physical activities. And this book can help you with the others. It's full of ideas that you may not have considered. By the time you've read this book, you'll be surprised at how few of your onefers can't be turned into twofers. Take a look at our example below.

Onefers	Twofers
Let the dog out	Take the dog for a walk
Carpool kids to school	
Get coffee	Walk to the coffee machine farthest from your office
Talk on phone	Stand up and do calf raises (see page 147) as you talk
Sit at computer	Do seated leg lifts (see page 142)
Go to lunch	Walk to a nearby restaurant
Sit at child's soccer practice	Walk around the soccer field while your child is playing
Mow yard	Push the mower instead of using the self-propelled feature

♡ *Be Adventurous*

Another part of creativity is the willingness to try new things. Sometimes they may seem strange or make you feel uncomfortable at first. For example, it may seem odd to do modified push-ups (see page 145) while you're waiting for your copies to come out of the photocopier. Or you might feel peculiar stretching your neck, arms, shoulders, and ankles on a plane.

People may wonder about you in the beginning, but don't let that bother you. Go against conventional wisdom. Be a physical activity trailblazer. Before you know it, people will see how it helped you and will want to follow in your path!

♡ *If the Shoe Fits . . . Walk in It*

As this book will show, you can fit in physical activity in hundreds of different ways. Most do not require any "equipment" other than your own body.

Walking is the most frequently mentioned aerobic activity in this book. That's because:

○ Everyone knows how to do it.

○ It's the most popular form of exercise.

○ You can do it anytime, anywhere, and with just about anyone or alone.

○ You don't have to change clothes.

○ It's fun.

○ The only equipment you need is comfortable shoes.

D **ID YOU KNOW . . .**
   In 1987, walking was first documented as the nation's leading exercise activity.

♡ *Walking and Working*

Ideally, you can wear walking shoes all day. But that's impractical in the working world. You can't stop every few minutes to change shoes, so the key is to wear comfortable dress shoes every day, all day. Choose shoes you can walk in for two minutes, ten minutes, or two hours. Can you imagine walking to the local deli for lunch in two-inch heels or tight loafers? Ouch! You'd probably call a cab for a ride back! And nothing will derail your fitness plans faster than pain.

Fortunately, that's just not necessary. Many shoe companies make dress shoes that have plenty of support and cushioning. Women should find the lowest heels they can. If flats are not appropriate for your business, try a low pump. Men should look for lace-up shoes. That way, you can adjust the tightness. When you find a style you like, stick with it. In some metropolitan areas, crisp business suits and sneakers (or Rollerblades) are the standard commuting attire. Remember, your feet should not hurt at the end of the day.

♡ *Weekend Workouts*

For longer sessions of walking—say, thirty-minute hikes on the weekends—it's a good idea to change into special athletic or walking shoes. They are typically more flexible, have special cushioning in the heel and the ball of the foot, and are more stable in the back part of the shoe. Use the tips below to help you select comfortable shoes for work or play.

*F*ITNESS BEFORE FASHION

These rules apply to both fashion and athletic shoes.

* Go shoe shopping when your feet are their biggest—after you've been on them all day.
* Wear the same type of stockings or socks that you will likely wear with the new shoes.
* Once the shoe is laced, make sure your longest toe is at least a thumbnail width from the end of the shoe.
* Stand on the ball of your foot. Do your toes have enough room to spread out? Does your heel come out the back of the shoe?
* Wear the shoes around the store for a few minutes. Be sure to walk on hard floors as well as carpeting. Do you notice any pinching, tightness, slipping, or rubbing?
* Don't buy a pair of shoes expecting them to feel better once you have broken them in. Make sure they are comfortable the moment you put them on.

D **ID YOU KNOW . . .**

Most athletic shoes lose their cushioning after 300 to 500 miles. How long will you own yours?

♡ *Wear Out, Don't Rust Out*

Now you know the benefits of being physically fit and active. We hope you've decided that whatever it takes, you want to leave that sedentary lifestyle behind. It's as easy as adding aerobic, strength-building, and stretching activities to your life, fitting them into your daily schedule wherever possible.

You'll need to measure your current fitness level. That's how you'll know later that you're improving. You'll also learn more mind games to help you make regular physical activity a habit for life.

Always remember, your body is designed to be active. If you don't keep it toned and active, chronic illness may cause it to rust out. As many healthy, active senior citizens say, "Better to wear out than rust out!"

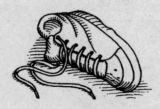

How Fit Am I?

Look closely at how active you are in a typical day. Do you routinely climb stairs, or is walking onto the elevator your exercise for the day? Do you take your dog for a run, or do you sit on a comfy window seat in your kitchen and watch him cavort in the backyard? Do you lift and carry heavy weights, or do you simply lift the telephone receiver to call the movers? What is your everyday fitness level right now? Take our simple test to find out. Circle the number that most closely ranks your comfort level for each activity.

OW DO I FEEL?

The Everyday Fitness Test

Aerobic Activities

After walking up a flight of stairs, I feel:

no discomfort   *short of breath*

    1   **2**   **3**   **4**   **5**

After walking from gate to gate in the airport, I feel:

no discomfort   *short of breath*

     1   **2**   **3**   **4**   **5**

After walking from one end of the mall to the other,
I feel:

no discomfort   *short of breath*

     1   **2**   **3**   **4**   **5**

Total aerobic points _____

Strength-Building Activities

After lifting or carrying heavy items (groceries, luggage),
I feel:

no discomfort   *weak*

    1   **2**   **3**   **4**   **5**

After pushing the vacuum cleaner or lawn mower, I feel:

no discomfort   *tired*

    1   **2**   **3**   **4**   **5**

After holding a small child for several minutes, I feel:

no discomfort   *tired*

    1   **2**   **3**   **4**   **5**

Total strength points _____

(box continued)

Stretching Activities

When bending to tie my shoes, I feel:
  no discomfort   *uncomfortable*
        1   2   3   4   5

When bending and stretching to make a bed, I feel:
  no discomfort   *uncomfortable*
        1   2   3   4   5

When reaching for the top cabinet shelf, I feel:
  no discomfort   *uncomfortable*
        1   2   3   4   5

Total stretching points _____

♡ *What's the Score?*

If your total score for any of the three fitness components was between 3 and 8, you're off to a good start. You can benefit even more by adding the "fitting in fitness" ideas in this book. If you scored between 9 and 15, you're in the right place. This book on lifestyle fitness tips and ideas will help you boost your fitness level. Then you can do these exercises (and more strenuous ones!) with ease and comfort. (For a more detailed assessment of your fitness level, see Appendix B.)

♡ *Playing It Safe*

Before you start making your life more active, be sure
you can do so safely. You'll probably find that the
activities we suggest in the following pages are easy
to do and completely safe. The only safety measures
you'll need are simply knowing your own limits and
using common sense. If, however, you haven't been
active on a regular basis for a year or longer and you
plan to start a *vigorous* fitness program, it's a good
idea to check with your doctor first.

D ID YOU KNOW . . .
      *One of the biggest reasons for giving up on
exercise is doing too much too soon.*

To be on the safe side, take a minute to fill out the
"Do I Need a Medical Okay?" checklist on page 33
before you start your program. It will help you decide
whether you should see your doctor before boosting
your physical activity level.

DO I NEED A MEDICAL OKAY?

Mark the items that apply to you.

_____ You have a heart condition and your doctor recommends only medically supervised physical activity.

_____ During or right after you exercise, you frequently have pains or pressure in the left or mid-chest area, left side of your neck, or left shoulder or arm.

_____ You have developed chest pain within the last month.

_____ You tend to lose consciousness or fall over because of dizziness.

_____ You feel extremely breathless after mild exertion.

_____ Your doctor recommended that you take medicine for high blood pressure or a heart condition.

_____ You have bone or joint problems.

_____ You have a medical condition or other physical reason not mentioned here that might need special attention in an exercise program (such as insulin-dependent diabetes).

_____ You are more than 25 to 30 pounds overweight.

_____ You are a man over the age of forty or a woman over the age of fifty, have not been physically active, and are planning a _vigorous_ exercise program.

Note: This checklist was developed from several sources, particularly the Physical Activity Readiness Questionnaire, British Columbia Ministry of Health, Department of National Health and Welfare, Canada (revised 1992).

If you didn't check any items on the checklist, you have the green light to become more active *slowly* and *sensibly*. If you checked one or more items on the list, visit with your doctor before increasing your activity level. He or she can help decide what is best for you. If you are more than 25 to 30 pounds overweight or if you are a man over forty years old or a woman over fifty, and if you've been inactive for years, you might call your doctor and ask whether she or he has *any* concerns about your starting a *moderate* activity program, such as walking.

♡ More Mind Games

Now you're cleared for takeoff, and you're ready to become more physically fit. The very fact that you're holding this book shows you're interested, but have you really made up your *mind*?

Couch potato habits are hard to break, and new habits can be even harder to adopt. Even when you're sure you want to change, you'll be more successful if you make these changes in *stages*. This is not just a mind game. "Curtain Call for Change" on page 35 lists the actual stages that each of us must go through in the process of changing. Which one best describes you?

CURTAIN CALL FOR CHANGE

Stage Fright—I have no desire to increase my activity level.

Stage Left—I think about the health benefits of regular activity and plan to change my habits.

Center Stage—I have been active but not on a regular basis.

Stage Right—I have increased my activity level and maintained it for a few months.

Encore—I have been active for several months and am certain that I can maintain my activity level in different situations.

If you're suffering from "Stage Fright," you're not alone. Hardly anyone starts on Broadway! As you read this book, begin to think about how some of the ideas and information could apply to you. Later, look at "Curtain Call for Change" again. By that time, you may have entered "Stage Left." Since you're holding a book called *Fitting in Fitness,* we'd bet that you've been cured of "Stage Fright" and are at least at "Stage Left."

If you are at "Stage Left," this book is the star-making script you've been waiting for. It's packed with tips and ideas on how to fit more physical activity into your day, routinely and almost effort-lessly. It also gives you a place to record your goals and help you plan and make changes in your daily routines. Remember: Start slowly and sensibly, but keep reaching for the stars.

If you're at "Center Stage," you'll find hundreds of ways to make all kinds of physical activity a regular part of your day. That's what fitting in fitness is all about. You're open to anything and ready to roll.

If you're at "Stage Right," you've hit the big time. Now you can make a great performance even better by learning different ways to maintain your activity level. And although you'll no doubt move on to "Encore" performances, you'll find yourself at "Stage Right" often. That's showbiz. But as you get more creative about fitting in fitness, you'll soon be back at the top of the charts.

If you've delivered an "Encore" performance, bravo! But don't throw away your script! Now it's time to "coach" someone else and add fun and new ideas to your repertoire. Then check out Chapter 9, "Fitting in Fitness When You Want to Do More." Of course, you'll also want to read the section on rewards in this chapter. You deserve them!

♡ *Checking Your Progress*

Now that you know how fit you are, how can you know that your fitness level is getting better during your weeks of fitting in fitness? The progress check in the box on page 37 is one way to tell.

O-IT-YOURSELF FITNESS PROGRESS CHECK

* Measure the time it takes you to walk 1 mile or some other specific distance.
* Walk the same course again after about a month.
* If you walk it faster, you've obviously improved!
* Record the dates and times of your progress checks.

♡ *Pieces of the Puzzle*

Of course, aerobic fitness is only part of the fitness puzzle. The other parts are flexibility and strength. Here are some ways to figure these measures of general fitness.

Bend and Stretch

Here's a simple approach for measuring your flexibility.

○ Sit on the floor with your legs stretched out in front of you.

○ *Walk* your fingers forward along the floor beside your legs. Do this very slowly.

○ Take note of how far you reached.

Did you make it much past your knees? Are you close to your ankles? As you become more active, you may become slightly more flexible, but it usually takes a targeted effort on your part. After you've tried some of our tips about how to fit in flexibility, take this simple test again. Are you any closer to your toes?

Strong-Arm (and Leg) Tactics

Take a minute to do the progress checks for upper body strength below. Then check your leg strength with the progress checks on page 39.

PPER BODY STRENGTH

Progress Checks

Wall Push

* Face the wall.
* Step out about 2 feet from the wall.
* Place your hands at shoulder height and about shoulder-width apart.
* Keep your body straight and bend your elbows until your face is about 2 inches from the wall.

Chair Push

* Sit in a sturdy chair with arms.
* Place your hands on the arms of the chair.
* Using your arms, lift yourself up from the chair.

How many times can you repeat either of these exercises? Try these again about a month after you've begun to fit in more activity. Can you do at least one more push or lift?

To test your leg strength, try one of the simple tests in the box below.

LEG STRENGTH

Progress Checks

Step Up

* Place your right foot on a step.
* Keeping your right foot in place, pull yourself onto the step. Avoid pushing with your left foot. It's okay to use a railing or a wall for balance if you need to.
* Step down. Then repeat this exercise with your left foot, using only its strength to pull yourself up.

Leg Lift

With this exercise, you'll need a big book, such as a dictionary, a telephone book, or an encyclopedia.

* While sitting in a chair, keep your feet together with your heels on the floor and with your toes lifted.
* Rest a book against your shins, balanced on your feet.
* Straighten your legs, lifting the book up.
* Lower your legs to the starting position.

How many times can you do the step-up activity
with your right leg? With your left leg? How many
repeats of the leg lift can you do now? Using the
same book as a weight, do these activities again in
about a month. Can you comfortably lift the book
more times?

Now that you know a few ways to measure your
progress, let's take a look at goal setting.

♡ *Ready, Set Goal!*

*"Say, Dad, can you spare a hundred bucks?" asked
John's son.*

*"Gee!" Dad sputtered. "Fifty cents, a dollar, even
five dollars I'm used to hearing. But what gives you
the gall to ask for a hundred dollars?"*

*The son responded seriously, "I believe in setting
my goals high."*

Well, we do, too, particularly in the areas of health
and fitness. In fact, setting aggressive goals is critical
to successfully fitting in fitness. Your goals need to
be exactly that, *your goals.* Try the following goal-
setting steps on for size.

Fitting in Fitness One Step at a Time

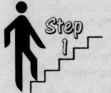

**Identify what you want to
achieve.**
What's important to you? Take a
look at the statements below and
choose which ones you value.

○ I want to feel better.

○ I want to have more energy to keep up with my family.

○ I want to spend less time watching television.

○ I want to begin an active hobby.

○ I want to improve my health.

○ I want to look better.

○ I want to lose a few pounds.

Step 2 Make your goals specific.

○ What do you want to accomplish?
Example: I want to have more energy to play with my children.

○ When do you want to reach your goal?
Example: By May, I want to be more energetic so we can enjoy some outdoor activities together.

○ How do you want to reach your goal?
Example: I will reach my goal by increasing my total daily walking time to thirty to forty minutes most days.

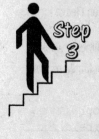

Step 3 Make your goals realistic.

Reaching your goals will motivate you, so make them attainable yet challenging. They should be well enough within reach that you will be successful. On the other hand, they should also present enough challenge to cause you to grow.

Goals for Today and Tomorrow

Be sure to set both short-term and long-range goals. Long-range goals take six to twelve months or longer to accomplish. Short-term goals are the stepping-stones of success that will motivate you to continue striving for your long-range goals.

Writing Down Your Goals

Here are some examples of long-range and short-term goals, along with space for you to list your own goals.

Examples of long-range goals:

- In one year, to be able to walk 4 miles without stopping.
- In six months, to have improved my fitness level enough to comfortably bicycle in the fall fund-raiser at work.

My own long-range goals are:

_____

_____

_____

Examples of short-term goals:

To climb the stairs at work when I arrive and when I leave for the day.

To walk my dog around the block at least three times a week.

To increase my time on the stationary cycle from fifteen to thirty minutes, two days a week.

My own short-term goals are:

_____

_____

_____

_____

_____

♡ *How Sweet It Is! Getting Your Just Rewards*

As you reach your goals, it will be important—and fun—to reward yourself. Your rewards don't have to be expensive, just things that are meaningful to you. Also consider how often you need to be rewarded in order to motivate yourself. Would you prefer recognizing your accomplishments weekly, as you achieve short-term goals, or monthly? Start by developing a list of rewards. Add your own favorite rewards to this list we started. Here are some wonderful ways to pat yourself on the back!

Rewards

Curl up with a new book	Schedule a massage
Take a relaxing bubble bath	Buy a sports watch
Visit or call an old friend	Buy a new pair of sneakers
_____	_____
_____	_____
_____	_____

♡ *Making Tracks, Keeping Track*

To track your progress, you'll need to record your fitting-in-fitness accomplishments. If you start having difficulty, you can look back at your records to remind yourself of past successes and what has worked for you. Also, you're more likely to accomplish your goals if you write them down.

The Physical Activity Diary in Appendix D of this book gives you a place to plan, monitor, and evaluate how you are fitting in fitness. It's essentially everything you need so you can prepare for successful change. You'll find places to log your daily activities, including the type of activity and the length of time you did it; keep a record of weekly goals; and list rewards. In the following chapters, you'll learn how to take advantage of many opportunities to fit in fitness.

♡ *Tips on Using Your Diary*

○ Carry your diary with you so you can immediately record your activity before you forget.

○ Use a star or some other symbol to indicate a new activity or an activity fit in at a new time. When you review your weekly activities, the new ones will be easy to find.

○ Record your comments about the tips that worked well for you. You may want to use them again.

You know your fitness level. You're ready with long- and short-term goals. And you're eager to reward yourself every step of the way. Well, like charity, fitness begins at home. In the next chapter, we'll show you dozens of ways to pack physical activity into life around the house. So have your vacuum standing by, get out Rover's leash, and keep the rake handy. We're ready to rock and roll.

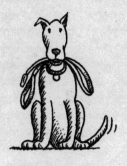

FITTING IN FITNESS AT HOME

Home, sweet home. You may not realize it, but home is a great place to fit in fitness. In fact, you'll find some real advantages to working in that workout right where you live:

○ You're already there. You don't spend time driving to a gym or recreational center.

○ You can fit in fitness when it's convenient. You don't need to juggle your schedule to fit fitness into your business hours or to fit in class times at a fitness center.

○ You can wear a faded T-shirt and mismatched socks if you want to—nobody will care!

○ Best of all, you can rack up twofers! As you do household tasks, you can work in a workout.

♡ *Home-Court Advantage*

Without even realizing it, you have your own "home gym," including:

○ **Aerobics classes**—offered at the most convenient times, every time you do laundry, vacuum, or mow the lawn

○ **Muscle-toning sessions**—available when you carry a sack of groceries, a basket of clothes, a garbage bag, or your child

○ **Flexibility exercises**—performed when you put on your shoes and socks or reach for the top shelf of your closet

So, how much time do you spend doing these activities every day? Start adding it up! You're already more active than you thought, right? Now it's time to add even more activity to your time at home.

♡ *Home Improvement*

Think of your average weekend. You're zipping around, trying to get things in shape. Take a few min- utes to get yourself in shape, too. The chart on page 48 shows you how to put some extra action into common household chores and routine tasks. When you think of other twofers, by all means, add them to the list.

THE BEST OF BOTH WORLDS

Routine Tasks	*Actively Improved Tasks*
Brushing your teeth	Stretch your legs as you brush.
	Do squats, lunges, calf raises, or the wall sit (see page 147) as you brush.
Making the bed	Increase the number of times you walk around the bed.
	Walk quickly or stretch farther across the bed.
Taking out the trash	Carry the trash can instead of rolling or dragging it.
	Carry less trash and make more trips.
Vacuuming	Really push and pull, switching hands to work both arms.
	Perform lunges as you walk with the vacuum.
Unloading groceries	Hold grocery bags, cans, bottles, or milk jugs in your hands; curl your hands, bending your arms at the elbows.

(box continued)

	Make more trips from the car into the house.
	Bend your knees to reach bottom shelves, stretch for top shelves.
Picking up and putting away	Make more trips, especially up or down the stairs.
Showering	Scrub the tub or shower, using a circular motion in both directions and alternating hands.

Get the picture? Now add some of your favorite music. To the right beat, vacuuming and bed-making can become aerobic activities! Go ahead and dance through your chores. It's a great way to put your best foot forward.

Sit and Get Fit

Yeah, *right*. As impossible as it may sound, you *can* actually add to your overall fitness when you're sitting down. (Okay, you have to get up for a few of them, but just for a minute!) Just use a little imagination. Take a look at the following ideas. They're easy and, after a while, almost automatic.

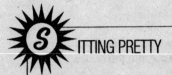

ITTING PRETTY

If you sit while . . .	You can be more active by . . .
watching television	stretching; squeezing a tennis ball to improve your grip; walking during commercials; doing push-ups, sit-ups, squats, or lunges
talking on the phone	stretching; doing arm curls or making rowing motions with a can of food in each hand; walking; doing squats or lunges; doing the wall sit
folding clothes	standing, then squatting or lunging to pick up clothes

For extra activities to do while sitting, refer to Appendix A.

Even though each of these activities may seem minor, they add up quickly! Remember that you just need thirty minutes of physical activity a day. If you can fit in fitness for ten minutes while watching commercials or talking on the phone, you'll need only one or two other activities to put you over the top. And you haven't left the house or had to wear spandex!

♡ *Outdoor Workouts*

Want to put some real muscle into your bid for fitness? Walk out the front door and into some serious physical activities. As you do the tasks listed below, look for chances to turn them into twofers. For instance, use a push mower and do lunges instead of using a power mower.

ALL IN A DAY'S WORKOUT

Wash/wax car
Mow lawn
Rake grass/leaves
Start a garden
Sweep the patio
  and walkways

Build a fence
Clean garage
Wash windows
Paint
Dig holes for shrubs or
  trees

Maybe you've been doing these chores all along without giving yourself credit for fitting in fitness. If so, add them to your daily count of physical activity. You may start looking at outdoor chores in a whole new way. See them as golden opportunities to stay fit and healthy—without paying health club prices!

Doggone Fitness

Looking for extra activities to boost your fitness level? You don't have to look farther than your own backyard. See Rover run. He runs because you let him outside. Next time, instead of just letting him run in the yard, take him for a walk. In time, you and Rover will have a regular routine that really racks up fitness points. Best of all, seeing him waiting so eagerly by the door will help you remember to fit in fitness.

Postage and Handling

Now take a look at your front yard. Instead of just walking to your mailbox, why not walk around the block first? Let getting your mail be a reminder to take a daily walk.

♡ *Love Thy Neighborhood*

Once you get out of your yard, you'll find dozens of ways to fit in fitness within your neighborhood. Some of the ideas listed below not only will give you fitness benefits but also will let you feel a sense of accomplishment and community. Consider volunteering for one or more of these community services:

○ Helping elderly neighbors maintain their yards and homes

○ Landscaping community properties

○ Participating in Adopt-a-Spot in your community (keeping a small piece of land litter-free or maintaining the flowers)

○ Helping your community plant trees, clean parks, or build playground structures

You probably have neighbors who are trying to fit in fitness, too. Go for a walk with one of them and brainstorm. You may think up specific ways to help make fitting in fitness easier. For example, in Chapter 6, "Fitting in Fitness with Kids," you'll learn how to start a neighborhood babysitting and fitness co-op.

Rallying the Troops

Make a point to scout around in your community. You might find that you live closer to parks, trails, or bike paths than you realized. Also, look for clubs or groups that meet to walk, run, or bicycle. Joining these groups is a great way to socialize with other people who share at least one similar interest (fitness!). Such groups also offer social support if you meet with them regularly.

As you can see, fitting in fitness at home is easy. The opportunities are everywhere. But what if you feel that you spend all your time at work? Not to worry. With some creativity and determination, you can work out at work every day. In the next chapter, we'll show you how to manage your day, help your cardiovascular system, and right-size your thighs.

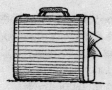

FITTING IN FITNESS AT WORK

Does it sometimes seem as though you spend every waking minute at work? You leave home at the crack of dawn and don't get back until after dark. Even if you work just a regular eight-hour day, plus commuting time, you often have very little time for anything but dinner and reading the paper. No wonder you claim you don't have time to exercise!

♡ Work As a Workout

In the old days, people got their workout on the job because the work itself was often hard physical labor. But with the onset of automation and more efficient technologies, much of today's work is no more strenuous than turning on a computer.

Some occupations still include regular physical activity. Mail carriers walk for hours. Bicycle couriers rack up a lot of miles. Many construction workers still dig, lift, and climb. If your job is strenuous, you probably don't need to spend extra time working out. You can still benefit from stretching and strength-building activities, however.

The rest of us, in mostly sedentary jobs, can fit in fitness at work. In fact, managing to work some physical activity into your workday can really make a difference in your health. One British study followed the employees of London's famous red double-decker buses. Each bus has a driver, who sits most of the day, and a conductor, who walks the aisles (upstairs and down) to collect fares. The researchers compared the health status of the sedentary drivers and the physically active conductors. The study found that the conductors had significantly lower rates of heart disease. Plus, of those who did have a heart attack, the conductors were more likely to survive than were the drivers.

In this chapter, we offer practical ideas for "working out" at work. Best of all, none of the ideas requires you to change clothes—or even loosen your tie!

Just for fun, we've also given you a few whimsical ideas for burning calories at work.

CORPORATE CALORIE COUNTING

Worksite Physical Activities	Calories Burned
Making a mountain out of a molehill	450
Passing the buck	25
Climbing the corporate ladder	275
Beating your head against the wall	65
Wading through paperwork	89
Balancing the budget	176
Jumping to conclusions	50
Fighting fires	389
Tooting your own horn	15
Beating around the bush	38

♡ *Office Politics*

Regardless of your occupation, you can probably take several short breaks during the day. Some companies even have wellness programs, including the use of fitness centers, that encourage employees to be physically active.

♡ *Heart At Work*

Find out whether your worksite offers the AHA Heart At Work program. If it doesn't, contact your local AHA affiliate. Ask whether someone can give a lunchtime talk to you and your co-workers. He or she can show you how to conduct a Heart At Work activity, such as the popular Adopt-a-Couch Potato.

♡ *Reengineering Your Workday*

Start by thinking about your typical workday. Do you have a set schedule? Are you required to be at your desk or workstation for certain periods during the day, or is each day different?

Whether you work twenty, forty, or sixty hours each week, rethink the way you spend your time. Be creative and inventive to fit in fitness. Here are a few examples:

○ *Arrive earlier.* Even five minutes earlier will help. This will give you time to park farther from the building. Leaving home earlier sometimes gives you the added benefit of less traffic and less time for your commute.

○ *Stay later.* Will leaving five minutes later really make that much difference in your child-care routine or other evening plans? Doing something physical for those few minutes will help you reach your thirty-minute goal. (It may even relax you so that the traffic won't seem so bothersome!) If you can walk or do some other physical activity for a little longer time, you might avoid the worst of the traffic and get home about the same time anyway.

○ *Give yourself a break.* Don't stay at your workstation for eight hours straight. At the very least, you need two fifteen-minute breaks during the day. So take five of those fifteen minutes to walk or do stretches. It'll re-energize you and add to your fitness level.

○ *Move during lunch.* Most people have thirty min-utes to an hour for lunch. But how much time does it really take to eat your lunch? What do you do with the rest of your lunchtime? Many people read, play cards, take a nap, or just sit around talking. "Sit" is the key word here! Why not use the extra time to be active? You can fit in a good ten- to twenty-minute walk before going back to work.

○ *It all adds up.* It's easy to get thirty minutes of physi-cal activity a day. All you need is five minutes before and after work, five minutes on your breaks, and ten minutes at lunch. Now *that's* efficiency—working all day and getting in a healthful workout, too!

♡ *Workout at Your Workstation*

If you're a teacher, factory line worker, or retail sales-person, you probably spend a lot of time on your feet. Though you get more physical activity than people who sit at a desk all day, it's usually not enough to gain health benefits. That's why it's important for you to find other ways to get moving!

The problem is that standing all day causes the blood to pool in your feet and legs. Then they begin to swell and hurt. If you can move around, your muscles contract often. That helps prevent this pooling by moving the blood through your veins and back to your heart. Standing for hours can also cause back strain, a major cause of absenteeism. If you take the time to stretch and move, you'll help relieve the strain and make your back stronger.

If you're a customer service representative, control room operator, or telephone salesperson, you sit in the same place all day except for brief breaks. On the other hand, if you're a manager, your time may be a little more flexible, but you still may spend a lot of time at your desk. Are you a truck driver, bus driver, or traveling salesperson? If you're driving, you have the biggest challenge of all. You won't be able to do many of the activities described in this chapter, so check out Chapter 5, "Fitting in Fitness on the Road." It may be just the ticket!

No matter what your workplace—a closed office, a cubicle, or an open work area—you can build physical activities into your regular work routine.

At first, when your co-workers see you pacing, stretching, and doing some of the other physical activities we suggest, they may question your sanity. If so, just show them this book. Before you know it, you'll have the whole office working out!

Desk Set

Let's start with activities you can do while sitting at your desk. For additional ideas, see Appendix A.

○ *Get a Grip.* Gently squeeze a soft tennis ball or other ball that provides some resistance. Repeat several times. This activity is good for strength-ening your grip. That can help when you play tennis or golf, rake leaves, or open jars.

○ ***Stretched to the Limit.*** Keep several sizes of heavy-duty rubber bands near your phone. (Smaller and thicker rubber bands will offer more resistance.) As you talk, do the following exercises:

□ Slip a rubber band over the fingers of both hands (don't include your thumbs). Put your hands together, palms facing each other. The rubber band should rest over the knuckles on both hands. Keeping your elbows at your sides, slowly pull your hands apart until you reach the rubber band's stretch limit. Slowly return to the starting position. Repeat four to eight times.

□ Put a large rubber band around one of your chair legs. Slip one foot into the rubber band. Position the rubber band on the front of your leg, at ankle height. Slowly extend your lower leg upward, pivoting at your knee until you reach the rubber band's stretch limit. Slowly return to the starting position. Repeat four to eight times for each leg.

𝒲ALKIE-TALKIE I

While you're on the phone, stand up and pace. Or get an extra-long phone cord so you can really stretch while you're walking. You may prefer a speakerphone or cordless phone or headset so that you can leave your office or workstation. Think how efficient you'll be if you can deliver a memo to a colleague two doors down while you're talking to a client on the phone!

♡ *Flex Time*

Here are some stretching activities that will relieve tension and improve flexibility:

○ ***Bytes.*** Looking straight ahead, open your mouth as wide as you can. Hold for ten seconds. Relax. Repeat several times.

○ ***Take a Bow.*** Make sure you have plenty of room in front of you. Reach both arms over your head. Slowly bend at the waist and lower your upper body down onto your lap. Keep your arms extended. Hold for five seconds. Slowly return to the upright position and hold for five seconds. Repeat the whole movement four to eight times.

○ ***Standing Ovation.*** Stand up and give yourself a big hand by extending your arms to your sides at shoulder height. With your palms facing each other, quickly bring your hands together in front of you. Return your arms to the starting position. Repeat the activity ten times.

○ ***The Wave.*** Stand up with your feet slightly apart (1 to 2 feet). Raise both arms over your head. Lean to the left, bending slightly at the waist. Stop as soon as you feel a slight stretch in your right side. Hold for ten seconds. Slowly straighten up. Repeat to the right side.

THE TWO-MINUTE TEST

Can't find time to do ten- or fifteen-minute walks at work? Then try two-minute walks instead. You can find dozens of opportunities for easy-to-do two-minute walks. Work in a walk before work, at your breaks, at lunch, and after work.

Not convinced? Then take this two-minute test. Get a watch with a second hand. Now briskly walk in your building for two minutes, looking periodically at the watch. Stop as soon as you hit two minutes.

Are you surprised how quickly two minutes passed? Look how much distance you covered! Now you know how far you have to go to fit in a quickie walk. It's amazing how quickly these two-minute walks add up.

♡ Send Yourself a Memo

Until fitness at work becomes a habit, you'll have to be creative about reminding yourself to get up and move around. Give these ideas a try:

○ *Write physical activity "appointments" into your daily planner or computer scheduler.* Respect them as you would any other appointment. Plan at least a week ahead so that you're not sidetracked by last-minute disruptions.

○ *Post notes in your workspace.* Try leaving yourself

little reminders that say, "Goal: two ten-minute walks today!" or "Move it or lose it!" or "Can I deliver a message instead of calling?" or whatever will help you fit activity in all day long. Put the notes in places you're likely to look at often—on your computer, phone, or calendar or on your office or cubicle door frame at eye level.

○ *Set a timer on your computer or your watch to remind you to get up every hour.* A quiet alarm clock or kitchen timer will work, too. Even if you don't get up and move each time the timer goes off, being reminded about doing some type of physical activity will help you make it a habit.

Record your activities and your progress in the diary on page 163. Jot progress notes in your daily planner. Some people develop their own computer spreadsheet just to keep track of their physical activities!

♡ *Have an Out-of-Office Experience*

Expand your workout options beyond your work-space without leaving your building. Try the following ideas:

○ *Management by Walking Around.* Visit people instead of calling them on the phone. Take longer routes to the rest room or to get coffee. Better yet, use the stairs to get to a rest room or coffee machine several floors above or below your work area.

○ *Photocopy Push-ups.* Do a few standing push-ups while waiting for your copying job to finish.

○ *Going Up?* Take the stairs instead of the elevator. Stop at every other floor and do a few calf raises on the landing.

ALKIE-TALKIE II

If you have one-on-one updates with colleagues, ask if they'd join you for a walk-and-talk business meeting.

OUR "HIDDEN AGENDA"

Sitting in meetings for hours can pretty much torpedo your fitness efforts. But don't give up. Put these discreet activities on your hidden agenda.

* Press the palms of your hands together as hard as you can. Hold for five to ten seconds, breathing normally. Repeat several times.
* Put your arms at your sides. With your hands open, press your palms on either side of your chair as hard as you can. Hold, breathe, and repeat.
* Place your hands under the table, palms facing up. Push up on the underside of the tabletop as hard as you can. Hold, breathe, and repeat.

(box continued)

* Drop your chin to your chest and hold for ten seconds. Relax and repeat.
* Tense, hold, and release the muscles in your buttocks. Then tense, hold, and release your right thigh. Repeat with left thigh. Repeat with both thighs at the same time.
* Drop something on the floor and stretch your lower back as you reach for what you dropped.

If you're leading a meeting, make a point of giving everyone five minutes to stand up and stretch at least once an hour.

Go the Distance

You can fit in a lot of fitness before work or during lunchtime simply by altering your routine slightly. Take a look at these ideas:

○ **Park 'n' Walk.** Instead of spending five minutes looking for a close-in parking space, go to the farthest spot. You won't have to fight over that one! One company gave its employees incentives to park in specially marked spaces the farthest distance from the building. Parking garages are great for long lunchtime walks because they're protected from the weather and you can get in some hill work!

○ **Bus Stops.** Get off several stops early and walk the rest of the way.

○ *Walk Before Work.* Before entering your building, walk around the entire block at least once. The distance around a city block is slightly less than half a mile.

○ *The Mall-Rat Shuffle.* Bad weather? No problem! Go to lunch at a nearby mall and walk around before eating. Even better, walk almost the entire break time, then pick up lunch to take back to work!

D ID YOU KNOW . . .

Dallas, Cincinnati, Minneapolis, and some other cities have tunnels or skywalks that link many downtown office buildings and hotels. These areas are great for workday walking because they protect you from weather extremes. Also, many bustle with activity during work hours, so you can feel safe. Check with your local chamber of commerce to find out whether your city has tunnels or skywalks near your workplace.

♡ *Walk Away with Fitness*

One of the best ways to stay active at work is to make sure you have plenty of support. That's why a walking club works perfectly. As you read this, it's likely that dozens of your fellow employees are interested in fitness, too. They just need someone—perhaps you—to get them organized!

Start by making your walking club flexible.

Encourage walkers of all fitness levels, from couch potato to race walker. Hold your walks at different times of the day (before work, after work, at lunchtime). Introduce people to local walking resources, such as parks, malls, or clubs.

ORKSITE WALKING CLUB

Getting started is as easy as 1-2-3.

1. Get three to five physically active co-workers to help you start the walking club. Ask other employees what they prefer in terms of frequency of meeting, time of day, previous walking experience, etc. You can do this through formal or informal surveys.

2. Sell! Sell! Sell! Advertise the who, what, when, where, and how of the club. Use lots of different promotional methods (employee newsletters, E-mail, voice mail). Exercise your brain to come up with promotional ideas!

3. Keep people interested by

*   Giving walkers a tracking card so they can log their walking time or mileage.

*   Rewarding participation. Recognize people when they attain certain milestones, such as their first 10 miles or five hours of walking.

*   Marking routes or distributing maps showing distances around the workplace.

*   Providing information on walking. You might set up brown-bag educational seminars or devise a list of walking resources in the community.

ᵂ ALKING WITH HEART

You and your co-workers can put your hearts and soles into a good cause. Help fight heart disease, America's number-one killer, by participating in the American Heart Walk, an annual fund-raising event for the American Heart Association. Here's your chance to make a difference while getting fit. Contact your local AHA affiliate or call 1-800-AHA-USA1 (1-800-242-8721) to register your company for the American Heart Walk event in your area.

Though you can't really turn work into play, you *can* take time out to fit a little play into your busy day. It not only helps break the routine and keep your attitude adjusted, it adds mightily to your total fitness count for the day!

If you travel on business, the next chapter will offer serious enlightenment for staying fit on the road. The tips count if you're on vacation, too.

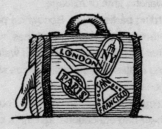

FITTING IN FITNESS ON THE ROAD

If you've been using travel as an excuse for not being active, you can give it up right now! With a little advance planning, you can turn life on the road into life in the fast lane.

The good news is that many hotels have fitness centers, jogging tracks, walking paths, and tennis courts. And many hotels and motels provide a swimming pool. Even if your hotel or motel doesn't offer these amenities, all you need is a good pair of walking shoes and some creativity.

♡ *Business Class*

When you travel on business, remember that the ideas in Chapter 4 are transferable. You can use

69

them at your client's office in Los Angeles as well as at your own office in Dubuque. You may have to be more aggressive and deliberate, but you can do it. Focus your activity toward one or two times during the day, perhaps before or after transacting your business. Why? We're just guessing, but we think you might feel awkward doing knee bends or calf raises in front of an important client!

♡ What's the Plan, Man?

When planning your trip, be sure to build in time for activity. Time spent being active is never wasted. Just remember the concept of planned inefficiencies.

♡ Break It Up

Most travel reservationists try to get you on the earliest possible connecting flight or train. Instead, ask how long it would be until the next-earliest departure. Maybe it would give you an hour or so to get in a good walk—and a good stretch.

If you're traveling by car, take an activity break every two to three hours. (See suggestions on pages 73–74.) Not only will it help with fitness, it will help keep you alert. With scheduled activity breaks, you'll have completed a full "workout" before you arrive at your final destination!

♡ *Best Seat in the House*

Reserve an aisle seat when traveling by train or plane. You'll have a lot more freedom to get up and move around. And you won't disturb your neighbors every time you want to stand up and stretch.

♡ *Pack It In*

If you take nothing else, pack comfortable shoes in your carry-on bag. Better yet, wear them until you get to your destination, then switch to dress shoes. You never know when a travel delay will give you the opportunity to fit in a brisk walk.

OUR FITNESS "READY BAG"

Take a tip from flight attendants. They keep a ready bag on hand, filled with everything they need for a trip. That way they don't have to pack all the essentials every time they head to work.

Likewise, keep a fitness ready bag handy. You'll automatically have what you need to fit in activity on any trip. From the list below, choose what will work best for you. We've left space for you to add any other items you might think of.

❑ 1 pair comfortable shoes
❑ Several pairs of socks

(box continued)

- ☐ Comfortable clothes (shorts, pants, and shirts of a quick-drying material)
- ☐ Plastic bags for dirty or wet clothes and shoes (you can also use the plastic laundry bag many hotels and motels provide)
- ☐ Pepper spray (for protection if you plan to walk outside the hotel)
- ☐ Jump rope
- ☐ Swimsuit
- ☐ Water shoes for pool walking (see page 79)
- ☐ Hand weights
- ☐ Ankle weights
- ☐ Exerbands or rubber tubing with handles
- ☐ Exercise videotapes
- ☐ Exercise audiotapes and cassette player
- ☐ This book (you'll find physical activities galore in Appendix A)
- ☐ _____
- ☐ _____
- ☐ _____
- ☐ _____
- ☐ _____

♡ *On the Road Again*

You've made all your plans. Your bags are packed. Now it's time to hit the road. Why wait until you arrive to fit in fitness? Let's start immediately.

Cars

If you're driving, you can't take your eyes off the road or your hands off the steering wheel. That's why frequent breaks are important. Take a fifteen-minute break every two or three hours. Find a park or rest stop and try these activities:

○ Walk briskly around the grounds.

○ Use the picnic benches for push-ups, chair dips, lunges, half squats, calf raises, etc.

○ Swing on the swings and teeter on the totter.

○ Thoroughly stretch your shoulders, back, and legs.

When you're on the road again and have stopped at a traffic light, take a few seconds to do the following activities:

○ **Window Stretch.** With your back firmly against the seat, extend your right arm toward the windshield. Hold for fifteen seconds. Move your extended arm across your body and reach for your side window. Change arms. Repeat, except reach with your left arm for the dashboard just below the rearview mirror.

○ **Modified Neck Roll.** *Keeping your eyes on the road ahead,* tilt your neck toward your right shoulder until you feel a slight stretch in the left side of your neck. Hold for fifteen seconds. Repeat on the other side. Do not tilt your head forward (you won't be able to see!) or backward (you may hurt your spine).

○ **Antsy Pants.** Shift around in your seat often. Otherwise, you restrict the circulation of blood to some muscles, causing discomfort, fatigue, and stiffness.

If you're a passenger, you can do these activities, plus some others in Appendix A, at any time.

♡ *Planes, Trains, and Buses*

There's not much room to play around with on mass transportation. Try, however, to get up and walk every hour or so, even if it's just to the restroom and back. You can also do the Modified Neck Roll, explained above.

In planes, you might be able to stretch your legs and back in the extra space near the flight galleys. In trains, you can stop between cars to stretch and do deep knee bends. Buses have almost no room for walking. Aside from standing up to stretch now and then, save your walking until you get to the frequent stops.

Try to loosen your lower back when you have a chance to stand. Here's an easy way:

○ Place your feet shoulder width apart. Bend your knees slightly.

○ Bend at the waist, keeping your back flat.

○ Rest your hands on your thighs. (For better balance, you can put one hand on a chair seat or a wall.)

○ Breathe out and arch your back. Hold for several seconds.

○ Roll back up slowly to a standing position.

*B*IN THERE, DONE THAT

Planes, trains, and buses don't provide much space, especially for your legs. And seatbelts are restrictive. Here's one activity you can do in your seat, though.

Keeping your lower back pressed against your seat, reach for the luggage bin over your head. First, alternate your arms, then reach with both arms at the same time.

If you're tall enough, push against the bottom of the bin.

ROUNDED AT THE AIRPORT?

Take Off on Fitness!

When waiting for a flight, most people sit and read, watch television, or people-watch. But not you. Before your flight or between flights, stretch your legs and fit in some serious activity. Here's how:

* Keep a pair of comfortable shoes and socks in your carry-on bag.

* Skip the moving walkways and courtesy carts— hoof it!

* If you're with friends or colleagues, ask them to watch your bags while you go for a walk. Be sure to allow them time for a walk, too. (Don't leave your bags unattended or with a kindly stranger. Because of today's strict security measures, your bags might be confiscated!)

* If you're traveling alone, locate a locker and stow your bags.

* If you *must* carry a bag, get one with wheels. This takes the load off your back. Then, as you walk, switch hands frequently so you don't overuse or strain one side. If you carry your luggage over your shoulder, be sure to change sides every two to three minutes. Do *not* lug really heavy baggage! The benefits of the physical activity are not worth the risk of straining your back.

"CURL UP" WITH A GOOD BOOK

Grab the heaviest book you have with you. Hold it in your right hand with your palm up. Keep your upper arm still. Bending at the elbow, curl the book back toward your right shoulder. Do this in slow, controlled motions. Repeat twenty times. Change hands and repeat twenty times. Repeat fifteen times with your right hand, then with your left. Now do ten repetitions with each arm. Finish off with five repetitions per arm.

♡ *Make Arrangements*

Try to choose a hotel or motel with access to a fitness facility or a nearby walking route. (For more information, see pages 78–79.) But regardless of where you stay, you'll find physical activity options almost everywhere. Some are more obvious than others. You'll need to experiment a little to discover what works best for you.

Hotels

Most hotels cater to the fitness interests of their guests. In fact, it's easier now than ever before to be active while you're out of town. To ensure that you get what you want:

○ Contact the person you are visiting and ask for the name of a hotel with fitness facilities or nearby walking routes.

○ Ask your travel agent to book you only in hotels with exercise facilities and a swimming pool.

○ Call the hotel directly. Although many hotels boast fitness amenities, they vary considerably. Ask:

☐ What equipment and services are offered in the fitness facility? Is the facility on-site? If not, how far away is it? Does the hotel have agreements with local health clubs?

☐ What is the surrounding area like? How safe is it to walk in the area near the hotel?

☐ Does the hotel offer a map of nearby walking routes?

☐ What are some other suggestions for getting physical activity while in that area? For instance, do nearby businesses rent in-line skates, bikes, or other activity equipment?

Consider a room above the fifth floor and take the stairs. Make sure that the stairwells are open (unlocked) and security monitored.

Motels

Motels don't usually have as many fitness amenities as hotels. That's no excuse! You can still find ways to stay active. Since most national motel chains have centralized reservations systems, you'll need to call the specific property directly to find out:

○ What is the area like around the motel (traffic, safety, parks, etc.)?

○ How far away is the nearest public school with a running track?

○ Is there a swimming pool?

○ Is there a park or health club nearby? (If so, ask for the phone number so you can call to get more information.)

♡ Pool Your Resources

Most hotel and motel pools are short, so lap swimming gets tedious quickly. Instead, try walking in the water. This will give you a good workout because water provides so much resistance. Just walk or jog back and forth across the pool in waist- or chest-deep water. If the pool bottom is rough, you may want to protect your feet by wearing socks or special water shoes.

For variety and an all-around workout, try these water activities:

○ Use your arms to help pull yourself through the water.

○ Practice half-squats, lunges, and other strength-building activities described in Appendix A.

○ Skip across the pool and walk backward on the return trip.

○ Hold on to the side of the pool and do the flutter kick.

♡ *Room and Bored?*

You're sitting in your hotel room with nothing to do.
You could watch television . . . eat from the room service menu . . . or be active! Here's how you can get
thirty minutes of physical activity *and* watch your
favorite TV show:

○ March or jog in place during the program. Add
   variety by kicking alternating feet forward, taking
   steps to the side, clapping your hands with the
   beat, etc.

○ During each commercial, do different strength or
   stretching activities. Check Appendix A for some
   ideas.

Be sure to do a few light activities before and after
your thirty-minute workout.

Remember that you don't have to do your thirty
minutes all at once. You can do strength and
stretching activities when you get up in the morning
and march or jog in the evening. Other options? Try
jumping rope, using hand weights, or working out
with exercise tubing or rubber bands (see pages 97
and 99 and Appendix A.)

Ⓐ MAT-TER OF FACT

To make your floor activities more comfortable, just double- or triple-fold the bedspread or
blanket and lay it on the floor. Instant exercise mat!

𝓃 AB A CAB

If you're using taxis to tool around town, try:

* Walking several blocks before hailing a cab
* Getting out several blocks before you reach your destination
* Asking the cabbie for ideas about places near your destination where you can fit in physical activity

♡ *Make Yourself at Home*

If you treat your time on the road just like you do at home, you'll find plenty of ways to fit in physical fitness. When you return home, you'll be ready and able to pick up your activity pattern just where you left off.

Whether you're on the road or at home, you'll really have a challenge fitting in fitness if you have children. Whether they're seven days or seventeen years old, kids need your nonstop attention. Rather than putting your fitness on hold for seventeen years, you may want to read the next chapter for our ideas on "Fitting in Fitness with Kids."

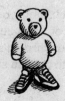

FITTING IN FITNESS WITH KIDS

Y ou need regular physical activity, and your children do, too! The sad truth is that today's children are more out of shape than ever in America's history. Too much TV, mountains of movies and video games, cutbacks in school athletic programs, and poor eating habits are contributing to a generation of out-of-shape kids, especially teenagers. If you want to help reverse this trend in your children, start today. You can't begin too early to raise fitness-minded kids.

If you have young children, you can fit in physical activities in hundreds of ways. Just use some imagination—yours and your children's. This chapter will give you some ideas to get you started.

♡ *Baby Talk*

So you have a new baby! Along with that angelic smile, petal-soft skin, and voracious appetite come more work for you, less sleep, and far less time for fitness. Fortunately, as your baby grows, you'll get more sleep and your energy level will rise. In the meantime, you and your baby can start fitting in fitness early.

JUST YOU AND ME, BABE

* Walk with your infant instead of rocking in a rocking chair.
* Hold your baby while sitting on the floor, then rock back and forth instead of using a rocking chair.
* While your infant's resting on a floor pad, do a few peekaboo push-ups or sit and stretch.

Is your baby ready for the great outdoors? Take him or her with you when you go for your walks. Push a stroller or baby carriage, or buy a front pack or backpack to carry your baby. You can also get baby joggers, newly designed bike seats for babies, and carts to pull behind bicycles. See Chapter 7, "Fitting in Fitness with Equipment," for details.

As your child becomes more mobile, so will you! You'll be up and down a lot, constantly chasing after him or her. Soon you'll have a "workout partner."

♡ *Look Who's Walking*

When your child begins to walk, your game of chase will move into overdrive. So take it to the streets, the park, or the local shopping center. Sometimes you'll

○ Walk slowly (and patiently!) at your child's pace.

○ Walk briskly as long as your child is content in a stroller.

○ Walk briskly to keep up with your child.

○ Bend, lift, carry, set down . . . bend, lift, carry, set down . . . You get the picture!

---

*D*ID YOU KNOW . . .

October is National Family Fitness Month. See what your community is doing to celebrate, or start your own family tradition.

♡ *Easy Rider*

When your child is learning to ride a tricycle or bicycle, you'll find yourself standing and waiting more often than moving. Take another look at the suggestions for fitness activities for home. Adjust some of them to fit your new situation. Remember twofers? While spending time with your small king or queen of the road, you can also

- ◆ Walk and do squats or lunges
- ◆ Pace back and forth
- ◆ Jog or march in place

- ◆ _____
- ◆ _____
- ◆ _____

Add your own ideas, and talk with other parents for theirs. See Appendix A for even more.

Consider starting a babysitting and fitness co-op in your neighborhood (see the box below). This will help you carve out a "fitness hour" that everyone can devote to physical activities. Each parent takes a turn watching the kids at his or her house.

OW TO START A BABYSITTING AND FITNESS CO-OP

1. Contact as many neighbors with babies and young children as possible. Explain the babysitting and fitness co-op and what it's designed to do. Make a list of interested people.

2. Hold a meeting to decide on the best day(s) and time(s) for the co-op to meet. For example, you may meet every Tuesday from 9:00 A.M. to 10:00 A.M.

3. Determine the number of children who will attend. You may need more than one parent to babysit when you meet.

4. Make a babysitting schedule that rotates through all the parents as babysitters.

5. Have each parent write down any specific information that a babysitter may need to know about

(box continued)

his or her child. Provide this information for all
members in the co-op.

6. Drop off your children at the assigned home, then
get moving!

A babysitting and fitness co-op eliminates a major
barrier to regular physical activity. It establishes a
specific time when you can fit in fitness. It also provides the social support of friendly neighbors. Social-
izing is good for your child, too.

♡ Child's Play

As your child grows older, play games that get both
of you physically active. You'll have some fun time
with your child, plus add some fitness points. Here
are some of our favorite childhood games. What are
yours?

Duck, Duck, Goose!   Mother, May I?
Red Light, Green Light   Scavenger Hunt (combined
                                  with a walk)

_____   _____

_____   _____

♡ *Singing the Spectator-Sports Blues*

As time marches on, your junior workout partner is likely to keep working out while you get involved in several new spectator sports. Why does this happen? Because you may not be interested in hanging on the monkey bars, and the coach might not want you on the ball field. It's easy to let yourself get sidelined.

If your child is on the team, follow the action. Walk around the playground, run along the sidelines, jog around the ball field. Use this time when you'd ordinarily sit in the bleachers to rack up fitness points.

♡ *Reading, Writing, and . . . Resting*

When budgets are tight, many physical education programs are cut. Many children go to P.E. classes just a few times a week, if at all. If your child is enrolled in child care or after-school care, make sure the program offers plenty of physical activities.

ID YOU KNOW . . .

  ✳ Research shows that physical activity
     declines dramatically with age during

(box continued)

> adolescence. Girls are even less active than
> boys.
> * Nearly half of young people ages 12 to 21 are
>   not vigorously active on a regular basis.
> * Among high school students, enrollment in
>   P.E. classes in recent years has dropped
>   from 42 percent to 25 percent.
> * Only 19 percent of all high school students
>   report being physically active for twenty min-
>   utes or more in daily P.E. classes.

Just how much activity is your child getting?
Here's an easy way to figure how your child's time is
being spent.

Activity Account

How many hours each week does your child

Sit in class?	_____
Watch television?	_____
Use a computer or play video games?	_____
Total number of inactive hours per week	_____
Participate in physical education classes?	_____
Play actively?	_____
Play organized sports?	_____
Dance?	_____
Total number of active hours per week	_____

Do the numbers surprise you? So what can you
and your child do to boost your activity levels? Begin

by setting a good example. If you're a classic couch potato, you'll probably produce little spuds. If your child is active, it's important for you to join in. You can't start too early to develop good fitness habits with your child. Encourage family fun and fitness with after-dinner walks, bicycle rides, or in-line skating. The more activities you introduce to your child, the better the chances of finding something he or she will enjoy enough to keep doing on a regular basis.

♡ *Activities That Run in the Family*

Create a list of activities, such as the one below, for your family to do. The key word here is active! Ask family members to help you add to the list.

◆ Go bowling.
◆ Plant a garden.
◆ Visit an amusement park.
◆ Go roller skating.
◆ _____
◆ _____

◆ Go ice skating.
◆ Go in-line skating.
◆ Rent a canoe.
◆ Go for a swim.
◆ Ride bikes.
◆ _____
◆ _____

◆ Take a hike.
◆ Pedal a paddle-boat.
◆ Walk the dog.
◆ Go square dancing.
◆ _____
◆ _____

ID YOU KNOW . . .

A short family walk or run is offered before most organized road races or walks. What an opportunity! Get involved in a community or charity event. You and your family may be inspired by the number of people who participate.

♡ *I Was a Teenage Couch Potato*

Surging hormones and physical inactivity are a disastrous combination. Like never before, your teenager needs regular physical activity. Ironically, today's teens rarely get it. In fact, though maturing physically, the typical teenager:

○ Gets limited physical activity at school

○ Isn't active in organized sports

○ Isn't interested in participating in family fitness activities

○ Drives instead of walks or bicycles for transportation

The fitness statistics for today's high school students compared with those of twenty-five years ago are pretty dismal. That why it's imperative to offer your teenager alternatives to life in the slow lane. Consider these fitness-related ideas:

○ Enroll your teen at a local gym or YMCA.

○ Suggest and encourage team sports. Offer to coach or sponsor a neighborhood, community, or other local team.

○ Suggest and encourage individual sports, such as walking, running, swimming, and biking.

○ Brainstorm with your teen on how to fit in fitness with friends. Suggest that they walk through the mall or go in-line skating.

○ Suggest an active part-time job. Officiating, waiting tables, and caddying all provide fitness opportunities.

○ Have your child earn car privileges or extra allowance through yard work or other physical activities.

○ Explain the importance of fitness, emphasizing looks as well as health. Teens want to be attractive to their peers!

○ Be a role model for physical activity. Point out others, such as famous athletes, who are physically active.

Keep your eyes and ears open for opportunities to encourage fitness, even if it's just a pick-up basketball game. Remember, kids develop habits early in life, so model good fitness habits now.

♡ *Traveling with Baby*

Infants tend to fall asleep during short car rides, but when you're traveling on longer trips, they become as restless as any adult. To make your baby's trip—and yours—more enjoyable, try these tips:

○ Ask a backseat passenger to move and massage your baby's arms and legs while the baby is in the car seat.

○ Pack a large blanket, and let your baby crawl on it during rest stops.

○ Help your baby walk around at rest stops.

○ After allowing your baby to get some activity, pick him or her up and walk around outside. You'll get a few minutes of activity, and your baby will enjoy the fresh air.

○ When traveling by plane, take your baby out of the babyseat for a short period. Help your child stand and stretch, just as you would.

♡ *Survival of the Fittest*

Don't think of long car trips as ordeals to try to survive. Instead, plan some activities to break the monotony. Try working on your child's fine motor skills. For that, you may need a few easy-to-bring items.

Stringing Along

What could be easier to carry with you than a piece of string or yarn about 18 to 20 inches long? That's all it takes for several games. Tie the ends of the string or yarn together. Now you can make the Eiffel Tower or Jacob's ladder. Take some extra string— these string games may be fun for all!

Music, Please!

Most children love to listen to audiotapes. Look for the ones with instructions for hand games. Check your local library and try them out.

Have a Ball

When you've played all the car games you can, it's time to pull over. Making frequent stops with kids will make traveling more enjoyable. Stop at rest areas, parks, or restaurants with a place for kids to play. If you're traveling by car, add the following items to your packing list:

○ Small ball—tennis ball, softball

○ Soccer ball

○ This book—to have tips on hand and your diary to record activity

○ _____

○ _____

♡ *Take a Hike*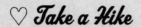

Watch for scenic roadside stops. They can offer a chance to take a short walk or hike. To keep your kids interested in walking, go on a scavenger hunt. Before leaving home, list some things to search for. Check the box below for several suggestions. Bring small bags to put the items in as they are found.

℞ OADSIDE SCAVENGER HUNT

Small twig	Penny
Yellow leaf	Bottle cap
Acorn or nut	_____
Rock smaller than a quarter	_____

Remember to get involved and play with your kids. It will make your trip more enjoyable and more comfortable, too.

♡ *Happy Landings*

Traveling by plane? When you're changing planes, take advantage of this time to stretch and move with your kids. Keep your kids moving through the airport with our Airport Scavenger Hunt (see page 95). Before leaving home, list the items on a card. Let your child check off each item he or she sees. After three items are checked, do the first activity under "What to Do." Then find three more items and do the next activity, and so on.

AIRPORT SCAVENGER HUNT

What to Find	**What to Do**
Someone carrying red luggage	____Stop and do 10 arm circles.
Someone carrying a camera	____Stop and do the calf stretch.
Someone wearing a Hawaiian shirt	____Stop and do 5 jumping jacks.
An off-duty pilot	
A water fountain	
A shoe shine station	
An off-duty flight attendant	
A telephone	
Someone using a laptop computer	

Although it's true that the only thing you need for fitness is a comfortable pair of walking shoes, why stop there? From dumbbells to mountain bikes, from jump ropes to hand weights, from pedometers to treadmills, a world of equipment beckons you to adventure. In the next chapter, "Fitting in Fitness with Equipment," we know you'll find something with your name on it.

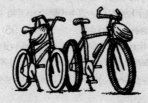

FITTING IN FITNESS WITH EQUIPMENT

W e'll say it again: All you need to fit in fitness is a comfortable pair of walking shoes. So why spend money on fitness equipment? In a word, *variety*.

Variety is not only the spice of life, it's what keeps physical activity *fun*. Boredom, on the other hand, is one of the most common reasons people give for quitting regular exercise. There's also the matter of balance. Equipment can help you acquire balanced fitness, including aerobic, strengthening, *and* flexibility activities. Finally, as your fitness level improves, you may move toward new fitness goals that require at least some equipment.

In this chapter, we'll suggest fitness "equipment" you probably already have around the house, as well as some you can buy. We can't possibly cover every type of fitness equipment, so we'll focus on the most popular ones.

♡ *Fitness "Equipment" on the Cheap*

Tired of walking for fitness? How about:

○ *Skipping Rope.* Reminds you of elementary school, doesn't it? The good news is that you're never too old for this classic favorite. Try it. You'll find it's still fun. Use heavy cotton or hemp rope. (Don't use nylon rope; it's too light and twists easily.) To measure for the right length, fold the rope in half. It should reach from your armpit to the floor.

○ *Bench Stepping.* Here's a step in the right direction. Start with a 3- to 6-inch step. You can use stairs or make a bench from bricks or cinder blocks and a sturdy board that's at least 12 inches wide and 3 feet long. Make sure the bench is totally secure. To vary your routine, check out a bench-stepping video to get ideas.

○ *Hill Climbing.* When you want to work out hard on a treadmill, you raise the elevation. This increases the intensity of the workout. You can accomplish the same thing for hundreds (even thousands!) of dollars less. Simply walk once or twice a week in a hilly area.

♡ *Throwing Your Weight Around*

You may not know it, but you have a "home gym," already stocked with all the "exercise equipment" you need. *Huh?* Sure! Take a look at the following "sophisticated" weight-training equipment:

○ *You Can Cancan.* Need a dumbbell? Try a can from your pantry. Use different-size cans for different weights. Just grab the nearest can and start lifting, curling, and pumping. If you complete twelve to twenty lifts or curls before you open each can, you'll be in great shape in no time.

○ *Cancan, Version 2.* Look in your garage for some empty paint cans with wire handles. Fill them with the desired amount of water or sand, and you'll have superb equipment for upper arm curls and bent-over rowing (see pages 138 and 144 for descriptions).

○ *Cancan, Version 3.* Don't toss those empty tennis ball cans, sports fans! Instead, fill them with sand, and seal the lid on with duct tape. Voilà! You have a dumbbell.

○ *Jug Jammin'.* Here's a unique recycling idea: Take a few empty half-gallon and gallon milk jugs and partially fill them with sand or water. They're ready to lift anytime!

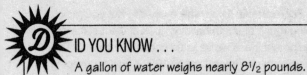

ID YOU KNOW . . .
A gallon of water weighs nearly 8¹/₂ pounds.

○ *Rubber Band Roundup.* Find as many kinds of stretchy rubber bands as you can—from a heavy-duty mailing band to a bicycle tire inner tube or cross sections of a truck tire inner tube. Then use them for resistance (see Appendix A for some activities). For an extra challenge, use more than one band at a time. Just be careful not to let them snap back in your face!

○ *Down the Tubes.* Go get those old athletic socks that are tucked away in your drawer. You know, the long tube socks that never stayed up. Fill plastic bags with sand, stuff them into the socks, and tie off the top. Now you have flexible weights you can lay across each ankle to add some resistance while doing leg kicks or leg lifts (see page 142 for descriptions).

♡ *Fitness Is in Store for You*

Before you even head for the store, ask yourself which of the three components of fitness—aerobic, strength-building, or stretching—you do the *least* regularly. Your answer will help you decide the type of equipment you need so you can add balance to your physical activity plan.

For example, if you walk every day but you're not doing much strength building, look at the resistance equipment ideas we've listed under "Equipment That Muscles In on Fitness" (page 109). If you're pumping iron but can't climb two flights of stairs without just about collapsing, check out our suggestions under "Equipment That Gives Your Heart a Workout" (page 103).

Now it's time to shop. The buying guidelines below will help you get the most for the money when you buy fitness equipment.

HEALTHY NUMBERS

From 1987 to 1994, the number of walkers increased 54 percent. Think that's impressive? Well, the number of people using treadmills rose a whopping 504 percent!

♡ Decisions, Decisions, Decisions

Here are some questions to ask yourself before making a purchase:

○ What type of equipment do you need?

○ What styles are available?

○ What do the different models cost?

○ What requirements (space, electrical, maintenance) does each piece of equipment have?

○ Where can you buy the equipment? (Retail stores, mail-order catalogs, garage sales, consignment shops, and classified ads are some options.)

○ What types of videotape do you need?

○ What kinds of equipment have fitness experts and your friends used? What did they like or dislike?

○ What would they recommend for your skill and interest level?

○ How are the different products rated in consumer magazines?

When possible, try before you buy. For instance:

○ Rent the item you're considering for at least three months.

○ Try out the equipment at a local health club.

○ Borrow a friend's equipment.

○ Try out the equipment in the store. Don't be bashful! Use it for more than a few minutes to get a real feel for whether it will work for you.

Don't forget to find out about the warranty and what you have to do if you need repairs.

○ Does the product have a warranty? What does it cover?

○ How do you maintain the equipment?

- How do you get it serviced? (For larger pieces of equipment, such as a treadmill, a repairperson may have to visit your home.)

- What does a service call or repair estimate cost?

C HECK IT OUT

Before buying home exercise equipment, check the safety features. That's especially important if you have children.

♡ Starting on a Good Note

Videotapes and Audiotapes

You don't want to try a new physical activity? Maybe that's because you don't know how to do it. Or you may feel intimidated in a crowded gym. High-quality instructional videos and audiotapes can teach you how to do a balanced workout—and you never even have to leave home!

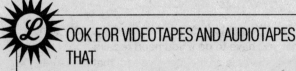

L OOK FOR VIDEOTAPES AND AUDIOTAPES THAT

* Cover the area of fitness (aerobic, strength, stretching) you want to learn.

(box continued)

* Are appropriate for your fitness level.
* Feature instructors who are certified by the American Council on Exercise, American College of Sports Medicine, Aerobics and Fitness Association of America, or Cooper Institute for Aerobics Research.
* Provide clear, easy-to-follow directions.
* Are less than five years old. (Fitness techniques have improved considerably in recent years.)

D ID YOU KNOW . . .

Listening to music while you exercise can help make it more fun! Therefore, you're more likely to exercise longer.

♡ *Equipment That Gives Your Heart a Workout*

Walk on the Wild Side—Pedometers

A pedometer is an inexpensive tool that measures the distance you walk. Clip it on clothing that has a belt or waistband (a pedometer usually is smaller than a beeper). Wear it all day to track how much activity you get in.

OOK FOR A PEDOMETER THAT

* Counts steps. Shoot for 10,000 steps per day. Increase your average number of steps as you become more fit. Ignore calorie readouts; they aren't reliable.
* Can be calibrated for your stride length. If you wear your pedometer all day, input an average stride length. If you wear it mostly for fitness walking, input a longer stride.
* Is electronic. But make sure the batteries are easy to replace.
* Has a sturdy clip for securing it to your clothing.

Wheeling and Dealing—Cycling

Today, there's a lot more to a bicycle than two wheels and a seat. You can choose from a host of different styles. *Touring bikes* are very lightweight and have narrow tires and curved-under handlebars. *Mountain bikes* have fat, knobby tires and upright handlebars. These two types are best for the serious fitness rider. *Hybrid bikes* have upright handlebars with narrower, less knobby tires. They are good for people who are less into long distances and daring downhill drops. *Tandems* (bicycles built for two) can be ridden only with a partner. *Cruisers* have upright handlebars, wider tires, a wider seat, fewer gears, and coaster brakes. They are good for people who just want to zip to the grocery store for a few items or wheel their way to work.

LOOK FOR A BIKE THAT

* ✳ Fits your cycling interests.
* ✳ Is the right size. Get an experienced cyclist or salesperson to show you how to properly fit a bike to your body size.
* ✳ Has fenders. Fenders will keep road splash from soiling your clothes.
* ✳ Has an adjustable seat and handlebars.
* ✳ Has only the gears and gadgets you need. You don't need twenty-one gears if you just want to tool around town.

DID YOU KNOW . . .

Biking is the third-most-popular fitness activity. Walking is number one, and swimming is number two.

Riding, Rain or Shine—Stationary Bikes

When rotten weather or a packed schedule keeps you off your two-wheeler, consider a stationary bike. Weighted flywheels or fans offer resistance as you pedal. To increase the intensity of your workout, increase the resistance on the flywheel or pedal faster. Have an outdoor bike you don't use? You can convert it to a stationary bike with a device called a wind trainer.

OOK FOR A STATIONARY BIKE THAT

- ✱ Has a comfortable seat.
- ✱ Is sturdy (that is, isn't wobbly).
- ✱ Has an adjustable seat height.
- ✱ Has adjustable resistance levels.
- ✱ Has a smooth-turning flywheel or resistance fan.

Do Tread on Me—Treadmills

For home exercise, Americans simply love treadmills. You can get a treadmill that is powered by your walking motion, but it will cause you to walk in an unnatural position. Motorized treadmills work best, but they're more expensive. Some treadmills have handlebars you can push and pull to get an upper body workout, too. On the downside, as a rule, you'll need to spend at least $500 to get a decent treadmill. Also, most treadmills take up a lot of floor space. If the garage is the only place with room for your treadmill, you probably won't use it.

OOK FOR A TREADMILL THAT

- ✱ Is sturdy.
- ✱ Has a wide belt that's long enough to accommodate your stride length.
- ✱ Has good shock absorption.

(box continued)

- ✳ Lets you vary your workout by adjusting elevation and speed.
- ✳ Has handrails down the sides.
- ✳ Isn't very noisy.
- ✳ Has a good warranty and service contract.

n OT ALL EXERCISE EQUIPMENT IS CREATED QUIETLY

From bicycles to treadmills, skiers to steppers, exercise equipment can cause noise pollution. Consider the noise factor when you buy home exercise equipment, especially if you plan to use it while others are sleeping or while you're watching TV.

Step-by-Step Fitness—Stair Steppers

Climbing stairs is a great cardiovascular workout. How can you climb stairs if you live in a one-story house? Get a stair stepper! They're relatively inexpensive and usually don't take up much room.

L OOK FOR A STAIR STEPPER THAT

 * Is sturdy.
 * Has pedals that move smoothly and independently of each other.
 * Has easily adjustable resistance.
 * Has a handgrip in front or along the sides so you can grab it for balance.

They're All the Rage—Exercise Riders

They're the new fitness phenomenon—exercise riders. Heavily advertised through infomercials, exercise riders are touted as strength-building aerobic workout machines. Do they work? Some do and some don't. Interestingly, price has nothing to do with it. Ask a qualified physical fitness professional to recommend a good exercise rider.

L OOK FOR AN EXERCISE RIDER THAT

 * Operates smoothly without jerks and hitches.
 * Has adjustable resistance settings. Even on the lowest setting, though, some are too hard for unfit people to use.
 * Has a comfortable seat.

***D*ID YOU KNOW . . .**

According to the National Sporting Goods Association, Americans bought more exercise riders than any other piece of exercise equipment in 1995. More than three million were sold!

♡ *Equipment That Muscles In on Fitness*

Tackle a Weighty Issue—Hand and Ankle Weights

Hand weights build strength in your arms, shoulders, and chest muscles. They also add resistance to arm movements, and the resistance burns more calories. You can use them while you're walking, watching TV, or talking to a client on the phone. You'll want to start with light weights and gradually build up to heavier weights.

***L*OOK FOR HAND WEIGHTS THAT**

* Have a smooth surface with no sharp edges. (A vinyl covering is a little softer on your hands than metal.)

(box continued)

* Have a comfortable grip that's neither too narrow nor too wide.
* Are well balanced in your hand.
* Are comfortable to use while walking. Look for hand weights that are easy to grip or to strap onto your hands. Start with a very light weight, just a few ounces, on short walks. You'll be surprised how tired your arms get! To get the full effect of the weights, be sure to pump your arms as you walk.

Ankle weights give your legs a workout. Unlike hand weights, ankle weights must be strapped on. Don't walk very far with ankle weights. They throw off your natural gait, and that can lead to injury. Instead, use them when doing leg kicks, leg lifts, or leg curls (see pages 142 and 146) while you're watching TV, talking on the phone, or working at the computer.

LOOK FOR ANKLE WEIGHTS THAT

* Feel comfortable; they shouldn't pinch or bind.
* Are easy to strap on. Velcro is usually better than strap and buckle types.
* Are adjustable so you can add more weight as desired.

♡ *Equipment That Has Flex Appeal*

Bounce Back to Fitness—Rubber Bands

Simple exercise rubber bands are inexpensive and easy to use. Just pull on the band—the more you pull, the more resistance you meet. Rubber bands vary in resistance from very light to extremely difficult. Since they weigh almost nothing, you can take them anywhere. And they're very easy to find. Most sporting goods stores carry them.

 OOK FOR RUBBER BAND DEVICES THAT

* Have handles. They put less strain on your hands than versions without handles.
* Come with an instruction guide that shows you how to do different activities.

Pump Iron—Weight Machines

Home gyms come in many shapes and sizes. They let you add strength-building and toning activities to your regular fitness routine. However, they do take up a lot of room. If you're aiming for moderate fitness, you don't need this type of equipment. It's mainly for those who want advanced muscular fitness.

LOOK FOR WEIGHT MACHINES THAT

* Are easy to assemble.
* Offer a wide selection of activities and weight levels.
* Are easy to switch from one exercise to another.
* Operate smoothly.
* Have clear operating instructions.
* Fit your body dimensions.

 Activity Is Where You Find It

Whether your exercise equipment is homemade or high tech, it can add variety and balance to your physical activity. Unfortunately, just having equipment in the house won't make you healthier, stronger, or leaner. You still have to do the work!

On the plus side, you don't have to depend only on your at-home workouts. In the next chapter, you'll learn how to fit in fitness while picking up your dry cleaning or taking your kids to the zoo. You know—fitting in fitness where you least expect to!

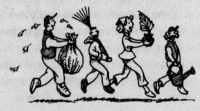

FITTING IN FITNESS WHERE YOU LEAST EXPECT TO

Think of your everyday life: running errands . . .
having family in for the holidays . . . volunteering in
your community . . . taking your kids to the zoo . . .
going to the dentist . . . doing all the little things that
fit into each day. You may not know it, but these
activities are ripe with opportunities to fit in fitness.

It's true. If you're going to the bank, consider
parking far from the door and walking in. Waiting at
the autobank is boring anyway. If you have family visiting for the holidays, why not go on a walk with
them? If you volunteer in the community, try to organize active ways to help out. And a visit to the zoo is
a fantastic opportunity to walk for miles and not even
feel it! When your dentist's receptionist tells you, "It'll
be a few minutes," tell her you'll be walking in the hall

or around the block. Turning onefers into twofers is
more fun than just sitting, right?

When you think about it, almost anything you do
can lead to an opportunity to fit in fitness and turn a
onefer into a twofer. You'll be astounded at the fitness points you'll quickly rack up. You might even
manage to "exercise" an hour a day this way!

♡ *Errands to Exercise By*

Okay, so you have to pick up your slacks from the
tailor . . . swing by the grocery . . . stop at the
cleaners . . . and go to the mall. You're in luck. You
can do all this and *exercise,* too.

At all your stops, park as far away as you can.
Instant perk: It's easy to find a parking space!
Depending on the number of stops you make, you
could accumulate ten to twenty minutes of walking
by the end of your errands! Take a look at the following ideas for more ways to pile up fitness points:

○ *Banking.* Get out of your car and go inside. Doing
   so can pay additional dividends over time because
   you'll get to know your banking staff personally.
   And vice versa. This relationship may prove helpful
   when you want to take out a loan or use other
   banking services.

○ *Cleaners.* Carry your laundry to and from the
   cleaners from across the parking lot. You'll burn
   more calories!

○ *Grocery Shopping.* Grab a cart on the way in. Walk around the periphery of the store at least once before heading down the aisles. Do some stretching activities while you're waiting to check out. Push your own groceries out to the car. Take the cart back to the store instead of leaving it in a corral in the parking lot. That will add a few extra walking minutes to your daily goal. All those steps add up!

○ *Carpooling.* What can you do with a carload of kids? Not much while you're driving. Park the car a few blocks from school and walk the rest of the way with them. After they go inside, take a couple of turns around the block, the school grounds, or the track.

○ *Hairdresser.* Do leg kicks and leg lifts (page 142) while you're sitting under the dryer.

○ *Shopping.* Be an "aerobic shopper." Walk the mall before starting your shopping. Climb the stairs instead of using the escalator. By fitting in fitness at the mall, you might not feel so guilty about "exercising" your credit cards.

♡ Does Fitness Run in Your Family?

At holiday time, physical fitness plans often get side-lined along with healthful eating. Think about it. You're

facing more stress and more calories than usual,
especially when Aunt Martha shows up with her world-
famous fudge and Grandma with her melt-in-your-
mouth divinity. Your only hope is to fight back with
stress-busting and calorie-burning physical activity.
Make it a tradition to work in some physical activity at
every holiday gathering. Here are a few ideas:

○ Be a part of an Independence Day parade. Join
  one in your community, or organize one in your
  neighborhood.

○ Organize a family turkey trot at Thanksgiving.
  Before or after the family feast (or both!), get
  people to get up and go out for a walk.

○ Try a snowman shuffle during the December holidays. Get everyone out for a brisk walk.

○ Go caroling. Map a route that covers your whole
  neighborhood.

○ Host an active holiday party. Invite guests to
  gather at your house. Then lead a walk (or jingle
  jog) through the neighborhood to view the lights
  and holiday decorations. (Tie jingle bells to your
  shoes for extra spirit.) When you return, serve a
  healthful supper of soup, hearty bread, and salad.

○ Organize an activity for your family reunion. Try a
  "fun walk," nature hike, scavenger hunt, volleyball
  game, or other physical activity. Make sure both
  young and old participate.

○ Take a walk with the neighborhood kids on Hal-
  loween. It'll be a real treat!

○ Go for a midnight walk, jog, or run on New Year's
Eve. Also, many walking/running clubs host New
Year's Day events.

♡ *Volunteer for Active Duty*

Giving your time and effort to a good cause makes
you feel terrific. And you can double dip by volunteering for activities that do your *body* good, too! For
example:

○ Participate in the American Heart Walk (held in
October in areas across the United States).

○ Clean up your street, a neighborhood park, or the
shoreline at a local beach or lake.

○ Do errands for others who can't get out of their
homes. (Don't forget the tips on page 52).

○ Help build or repair a house for a disadvantaged
family.

○ Coach a youth or adult sports team. And don't just
be a sideline coach. Do all the exercises you ask
your players to do.

Check with your local PTA to see whether it might
build a walking/biking trail for your school. Many
state departments of parks and recreation, as well as
transportation departments, have funds for community development.

♡ Take Your Show on the Road

When you want some entertainment, think "fitting in fitness." How? Some places you might go for entertainment naturally involve walking. For example:

○ Zoos

○ Arboretums

○ Theme parks

○ Museums

○ Monuments and historic parks

To get the most physical activity at each of these places, start by parking in the far corner of the parking lot. Once inside, map a route that has you crisscrossing the entire venue several times. This plan means you'll have to walk a bit between each exhibit. Remember our discussion about planned inefficiencies? It's not "inefficient" to fit in fitness while you enjoy a day at the zoo.

SPORTS FAN'S WORKOUT

Don't wait until the seventh inning to get up and stretch! Climb some stairs or march in place at least every quarter, every period, or every other inning. Better yet, add some activity at every station break.

♡ Take Your Name Off the Waiting List

So much of life is hurry up and wait. You hurry to the doctor's office, only to wait in the reception area. You race to a concert, which starts late. You wait in line to renew your driver's license. And on and on. Here are some typical hurry-up-and-wait venues:

○ Doctors' and dentists' offices

○ Restaurants

○ Concerts, theater, and other performance arts events

○ Bureaucratic offices

Get a new game plan. The next time you have to wait, ask how long the delay will be. Then walk around the building during that time. Find the stairs and walk up several flights. If you're stuck standing in line, do some stretching activities.

℘ REVENTIVE MEDICINE

When you're visiting a friend or loved one in the hospital, you usually sit and wait for hours at a time. All that waiting, plus the tension of worrying, can make you want to climb the walls. So climb the stairs instead. Or go for a walk. You need a tension releaser. Just let the nurses know where you'll be, then take an activity break.

♡ *An Added Routine*

From attending religious services to dining with friends or joining them at a movie, do you have certain activities you enjoy weekly? If you live close enough to do so, walk to your place of worship, the restaurant, or the movie theater. Or organize your friends to join you for a walk and a picnic at a local park.

Many places of worship offer fitness classes. If yours does, check them out. If yours doesn't, contact the program committee chairperson and offer to get a program started.

When you get into the habit of fitting in fitness where you least expect to, you'll quickly amass fitness points. But a day may come when even *that* isn't enough. If so, you'll want to explore the next chapter, "Fitting in Fitness When You Want to Do More." The hobbies, sports, and other activities we suggest can help boost you to a whole new fitness level.

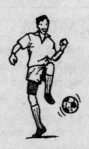

Fitting in Fitness When You Want to Do More

9

By now you're an expert at fitting fitness into your thinking—and your lifestyle. A little walking here, a little weight training there. You like having more energy, losing weight more easily, feeling better. The bottom line is that you *like* being active and you want to do *more*.

No problem! In this chapter, we'll show you dozens of fun ways to pack your life with physical activity. They might take a little effort and commitment, but the results are definitely worthwhile!

♡ Line Up an Active Hobby

When you look for a new hobby, consider one that's physically active. The hobbies listed below will give you hours of fun and fitness every week!

○ *Dancing.* Whether it's line, square, ballroom, tap, or some other kind of dancing, it's fun, it's social, and it burns calories.

○ *Gardening.* Ever envy people with beautiful yards, lush flower gardens, and fresh vegetables by the bushelful? If you have a hands-on approach to gardening, you'll burn calories galore—and have plenty to show for it!

○ *Woodworking.* If you do your sawing and sanding by hand, you can get quite a workout.

○ *Mushroom Hunting.* Don't take the most direct route. Hike a while before and after your find.

ART-TIME PAYOFFS

Want to stay fit while making a little extra cash? Consider the following possibilities:

* Usher at theater, concert, or sporting events.
* Sell souvenirs in the stands at the ballpark (now there's a workout!).
* Caddie (for a golfer who walks).
* Courier packages and letters around town by bike (or, if driving, park away from your destinations).
* Officiate at football, basketball, soccer, or hockey games. (Baseball, softball, and tennis officiating are not as active.)

♡ *Join the Club!*

Look in the local paper for groups that meet to:

○ Walk

○ Run/jog

○ Cycle

○ Hike

○ Dance

○ Canoe/row

○ In-line skate

Group activities are excellent because you're likely to find someone at your fitness and skill level. Also, you'll be around experienced people who can help you learn new skills. When you get to know people in the group, the activity will seem more like a party than a workout! And the icing on the cake: Many of these groups sponsor special events that benefit local charities, so you can look good and feel good, too!

p LAY TO YOUR HEART'S CONTENT

Keep exercise playful! Learn a new sport or activity with your family or a friend. Or return to some backyard favorites, such as croquet or badminton. Bocce, which is a lot like lawn bowling, is becoming more popular. Give it a try!

♡ *Give Yourself a Sporting Chance*

A great way to meet people and make friends is to join a sports team. You don't have to be a jock—just show up ready to play with enthusiasm. Though you can do some of these alone, they're a lot more fun in a group:

○ **Water Sports.** Swimming, snorkeling, scuba diving, canoeing, kayaking, skiiing, rowing.

○ **Winter Sports.** Downhill or cross-country (the best aerobic conditioning sport around!) skiing, snow-shoeing, skating.

○ **Racket Sports.** Tennis, racquetball, squash, badminton, table tennis (yes, it's active!).

○ **Dancing.** Country western, line, folk, ballroom, square, contra, ballet, tap, jazz, and disco (it's making a comeback).

○ **Team Sports.** Basketball, soccer, volleyball, hockey.

○ **Orienteering.** A hiking adventure in which you navigate your way through forests to designated checkpoints. You can compete against the clock or just enjoy the challenge and the scenery.

○ **Polo.** The horse isn't the only one getting a workout!

If you want to compete in a chosen sport, check into local leagues or master's groups. Master's sports provide training and competition for people fifty to ninety-plus years old.

♡ *Get Some R and R*

What's your ideal vacation? For many, it's lying on a beach. But if you crave relaxation and rejuvenation, try an active vacation. Exercise relieves stress and keeps your body fit and younger looking.

Hit the Slopes . . . the Trail . . . the Deck . . .

You can fit in fitness on most types of vacations. Just build in some physical activity on most days. For example:

○ Walk along the beach instead of just *lying* on it. Swim and play in the water.

○ Hike the trails at a state or national park instead of just driving through. Experience the natural beauty; don't just view it through your car windows.

○ Walk the golf course instead of using a cart.

○ On cruises, swim in the pools and at the beaches. Walk around the deck, use the exercise room, or take aerobics classes on the ship. In port, be sure to see the sights on foot.

○ Check out the lay of the land in a new area by hoofing it. Go slowly enough to really soak in the history, sights, and sounds. By walking, you can follow your own schedule, not that of a tour driver. Contact the area's chamber of commerce, historical society, or visitors' bureau for information on walking tours. Many guidebooks also suggest walking routes.

Move Over, Indiana Jones

"Adventure vacations" are the hottest segment of the travel industry. Try on these adventures for size:

○ Bicycling tour in New England

○ Hiking down and back up the Grand Canyon

○ Hiking to the top of a 14,000-foot (or higher) peak in Colorado (There are fifty-five to choose from!)

○ Canoeing on the lakes in Minnesota

○ Hiking the Appalachian Trail

○ Driving a herd of cattle to new grazing land on a dude ranch

For even more exotic ideas, hook up with a travel agent or tour company that specializes in active vacations. You'll find they offer trips for people, including families, of all ages and abilities.

Here I Am at Camp Granada . . .

Singing around the campfire . . . toasting marshmallows . . . gazing at the stars. That's what comes to mind when we think of camp. But that was then, and this is now. Today's summer camps are getaway vacations built around activities. Try a family camp over a holiday weekend. Or book time at a camp designed just for learning (or perfecting) certain skills. You can find camps for

- Bicycling
- Volleyball
- Skiing (downhill and cross-country)
- Running
- Golfing
- Fly-fishing
- Strength training
- Kayaking
- Hiking
- Horseback riding
- Snorkeling/scuba diving
- Mountain climbing
- Dancing
- In-line skating
- Surfing

Rank beginner or seasoned pro, you'll love a fitness camp. All you need is a willingness to learn and have fun! For details, read exercise-oriented magazines or ask your travel agent.

♡ The Perks of Health Club Membership

Okay, we confess. This is the opposite of "fitting in fitness." But after a while you'll find that fitness is somewhat addictive. As you begin to look and feel better, you may want to do *more*. That's where a health club comes in handy. It has the resources you need to help you attain higher and higher fitness goals. Plus, the support and encouragement from the staff and the other members tend to spur you on to being even more active than you may be on your own.

Every health club is different, but they usually fall into the three categories described below. In general, the more you pay, the more you get. It's important to visit all three types of center in your community to find out which works best for you.

○ *High End.* These full-service clubs have high-tech equipment and plenty of professional staff to help with personalized programs. They also offer a wide variety of classes and programs. Many provide extra amenities, such as child care, juice and snack bars, massage services, and a pro shop.

○ *Mid-range.* These centers have lots of equipment and a good variety of exercise classes. However, they usually employ fewer professional staff than their high-end counterparts. Also, they may not provide facilities such as a pool or walking/running track or offer extra amenities.

○ *Basic.* These centers have some equipment but generally don't employ full-time professional staff. They usually offer a wide variety of recreational sports leagues, such as basketball and softball. Examples are community recreation centers.

CLUB CRITERIA CHECKLIST

Visit at least one club of each of the three types. Then use this checklist to help you evaluate them to find the right "fit."

☐ Is the club close to your home or work? (Convenience is the key to being consistent!)

☐ Do its hours of operation and class times fit into your schedule? (You're not going to make a 5:30 P.M. aerobics class if you don't get off work until 6:00 P.M.!)

☐ Is it crowded during the hours you're likely to use it? Are there lines to use the equipment? Are the classes overcrowded? (Be sure to visit during these times and see for yourself.)

☐ Are the equipment, programs, leagues, activities, and classes ones that you enjoy or might like to try?

☐ Is the facility well lighted and well ventilated?

☐ Is the locker room clean and well maintained?

☐ What are the qualifications and certifications of the fitness staff? (Ask to see biographies or résumés of the staff.)

☐ Are staff or instructors available for one-on-one instruction? What is the cost? (This is especially important if you want to learn a new skill or perfect a technique.)

(box continued)

☐ Is it necessary to get a health screening before joining? (This is a good idea because it can identify preexisting health problems, such as high blood pressure. It can also establish a fitness starting point and help you set goals for improvement.)

☐ Can you get a trial membership to see whether a health club is truly what you need and want? Even a one-week or one-month membership can help you decide.

☐ What are the fees and payment plan? (Be wary of long-term contracts and pushy salespeople.)

♡ The More the Merrier

From line dancing to golf, gardening to pumping iron, a universe of activities can give you that adrenaline rush of fun while you fit in fitness. In the next chapter, we'll cover how to put it all together into a habit that will give you a lifetime of fitness and health.

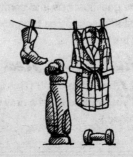

Putting It All Together

A s you've read this book, you've learned that there's no mystery to achieving fitness. It's easy to get fit and stay that way. You don't need a fancy gym or hours each day to work out. You simply need to fit fitness into your everyday life. Your new lifestyle approach to fitness will help keep your heart healthy for a lifetime.

♡ Launching Your New Lifestyle

The next few pages discuss six easy steps to help you launch your new fitness lifestyle.

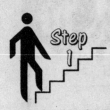

Make up your mind.

The first part of changing any habit is to think about it. For example, since starting this book, have you caught yourself on the telephone thinking, "I could do a few squats as I talk"? Or have you let your dog out and thought, "Rover and I could go for a walk"? If so, congratulations! You've already taken the first step.

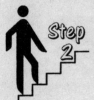

Create your personal fitness plan.

Start simply. You don't have to use all the fitness tips you've learned at once. You just need to

○ Select one or two fitting in fitness activities for the next week.

○ Record each activity in your diary soon after completing it.

○ Reward yourself for your accomplishments.

○ Stick with the activities that fit your lifestyle, then add another one next week.

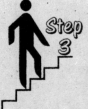

Include family, friends, and co-workers.

Let the people around you know what you're doing. Ask for their support. That will make your new lifestyle changes much easier. Invite them to join you and make some changes of their own!

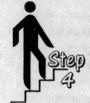

Track your new fitness level.
Repeat the fitness level checks outlined in Chapter 2 *often.* When you start to see regular progress, you'll be excited—and motivated to do even more!

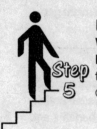

Keep moving forward.
When you have a relapse of old, inactive habits—and you almost certainly will—try the following rescue tactics:

○ Read your exercise diary to remind yourself of the activities that easily fit into your life.

○ Reread a chapter in this book for new ideas.

○ Stick reminder notes on your telephone, computer, or television.

○ Most of all, keep *Fitting in Fitness* close at hand!

THE FIVE R'S OF FITTING IN FITNESS
Keep this book with you to

✳ Refresh your memory. If offers hundreds of fitness activities to choose from!

✳ Refer to descriptions of specific exercises (see Appendix A). That will help convince you to try them.

(box continued)

* Remind yourself of your goals and the sweet rewards that follow. That's motivating!
* Record your activity. See how far you've come.
* Respond to curious looks. Did anyone stare while your curled a milk jug? Just show the lookers this book. Who knows? You might get someone to join you!

Focus on the paybacks.

Even short bouts of physical activity will help you net health benefits and burn calories. If you want to drop a few pounds, look at the chart below to learn the potential weight loss you can expect in a year simply from fitting in fitness.

Activity	Minutes	Days/Week	Pounds Lost per Year for Given Weight		
			130 lb.	150 lb.	180 lb.
Washing car	30	1	2.0	2.5	3.0
Grocery shopping	30	1	1.5	1.75	2.25
Playing with children (while standing)	20	7	6.0	6.5	8.0
Walking upstairs	6	5	3.5	4.0	5.0
Pushing a stroller	10	3	1.0	1.25	1.5
Walking the dog	15	5	4.0	4.5	5.25
Lifting light weights	10	4	1.75	2.0	2.5
		Total pounds lost	19.75	22.5	27.5

Wow! Hard to believe, isn't it? And you can drop those extra pounds without a personal trainer, fancy gym, or strict diet. You get all this, plus the heart-protecting benefits of regular exercise. It's all part of your new lifestyle of fitting in fitness.

We wish you good luck, good health, and a heart that lasts a lifetime.

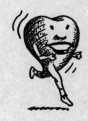

Activities for Total Fitness

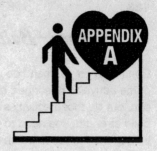

Aerobic, flexibility, and strength-building activities—all are needed for total fitness. Use the activities in this appendix to supplement the ones you've read about throughout *Fitting in Fitness*.

♡ *Aerobic Activities*

There are many aerobic activities. But when it comes to fitting in fitness, walking is clearly the easiest and most popular choice. Other favorites include jogging, biking, and dancing. Some beneficial choices around the house are vacuuming, washing windows, gardening, and raking leaves.

♡ Strength-Building Activities

Don't worry if you can't do more than a few of each of the activities described below. Just do what you can, but do those activities regularly. You see, to build strength, you need to challenge your muscles. In response to repeated challenges, the muscles will get stronger. As you become stronger, you may want to add light hand or ankle weights for added resistance.

When doing these activities, be sure to use slow, controlled movements. Also, remember not to restrict your breathing at any time when you are doing the activities.

Seated Activities

Make sure your chair is secure and won't roll while you do these activities.

Arm Curl

○ Sit toward the front of your chair with your legs slightly apart.

○ Grasp a heavy object (makeshift weight, paper-weight, book) in your right hand.

○ Rest your left hand on your left thigh.

○ Brace your right elbow against the inside of your right knee.

○ With your palm facing up and your elbow bent, slowly raise the object toward your right shoulder.

○ Repeat 12 to 20 times.

○ Repeat with left arm.

With Exercise Tubing (or large rubber bands tied together)

○ Sit as described above. Don't grasp a heavy object, though.

○ Instead, hold one end of the tubing in your right hand and hold down the other end with your right heel.

○ Bend your elbow.

○ Slowly raise your right hand toward your right shoulder.

○ Repeat 12 to 20 times.

○ Repeat with the left arm, holding down the exercise tubing with your left heel.

Arm Extension with Exercise Tubing (or large rubber band)

○ Sit with your back firmly against the back of your chair.

○ Hold one end of the tubing (or rubber band) in each hand.

○ Place your left hand on your right shoulder.

○ With your right elbow bent and your upper arm parallel to the floor, place your right hand near your shoulder, palm facing upward.

○ Straighten your elbow, keeping your upper arm stationary, until your right palm is facing the floor.

○ Move your right hand and lower arm back toward your shoulder.

○ Repeat 12 to 20 times.

○ Repeat exercise with your left arm, holding the tubing (or rubber band) at your left shoulder with your right hand.

Side Arm Raise

○ Sit with your back firmly against the back of your chair.

○ Hold a heavy object (makeshift weight, paperweight, book) in your right hand.

○ Let your right arm hang loosely at your side.

○ With your palm facing inward and your arm straight, lift and lower your entire arm to shoulder height 12 to 20 times.

○ Repeat with your left arm.

○ Variation: Lift the weight straight in front of you 12 to 20 times with each arm.

With Exercise Tubing (or large rubber bands linked together)

○ Take the same position as described above, but don't hold a heavy object.

○ Instead, with exercise tubing running underneath the seat of the chair, hold one end in each hand.

○ Keep your left hand in place as you move your right arm from your side to shoulder height and back to your side.

○ Repeat 12 to 20 times.

○ Repeat with your left arm, keeping your right arm at your side.

Punching Bag

○ Extend both arms horizontally in front of you.

○ Start punching the air directly in front of you, alternating arms.

○ Repeat 15 times with each arm.

○ While still punching, lower your arms and punch the air near your knees.

○ Repeat about 15 times with each arm.

○ Raise your arms and punch the air in front of you again, 15 times per arm.

○ Slowly raise your arms over your head and repeat the punching for 15 times per arm.

○ Lower your arms to the horizontal position again and do a final set of 15 punches with each arm.

Sitting Crunch

○ Sit with your lower back firmly against the back of your chair.

○ Put your feet together and bring your heels close to the front legs of the chair.

○ Grasp the front of the seat, near your knees.

○ Keeping your knees bent, slowly lift your right leg off the ground and then lower it without touching the floor. Keep your lower back pressed against the chair.

○ Repeat 12 to 20 times.

○ Switch legs and repeat.

○ Now put your feet together and lift both legs at the same time.

○ Repeat 4 to 8 times.

Leg Kick

○ Sit with your back firmly against the back of your chair.

○ With both feet flat on the floor, point your right toes upward.

○ Slowly straighten your right leg.

○ Raise your leg until it's parallel to the floor.

○ Bend your knee and lower your leg slowly without letting your foot touch the floor.

○ Repeat 12 to 20 times.

○ Repeat with left leg.

Leg Lifts

○ Sit with your back firmly against the back of your chair. Put both feet flat on the floor.

○ Point your right toes upward and slowly straighten your right leg.

○ Keeping your leg straight and moving from your right hip, slowly raise and lower your right leg off the chair 12 to 20 times.

○ Repeat with left leg.

Standing Activities

If possible, remove your shoes, especially if you're wearing high heels, to do these activities.

Remember to keep your knees very slightly bent. Locking your knees in a straight position could increase your risk of injury.

Upper Arm Extension

○ Hold a heavy item (makeshift weight, paperweight, book) in your right hand. Keep your palm facing your side. Let your right arm relax at your side.

○ Keeping your right arm straight, extend it behind you.

○ Bend *only* at your elbow, keeping your upper arm slightly behind you. Slowly bring your right hand forward, toward your shoulder. Hold for one second.

○ Return your hand to the starting position.

○ Repeat 12 to 20 times.

○ Repeat with your left arm.

Upright Row

○ Stand with your feet slightly apart and your knees slightly bent.

○ Hold a heavy object (makeshift weight, paper-weight, book) in each hand.

○ With palms facing back, pull the objects up toward your chin in a rowing motion. Be sure to raise your upper arms until they are parallel with the floor.

○ Lower hands slowly.

○ Repeat 12 to 20 times.

One-Arm Bent-Over Row

○ Hold a heavy object (makeshift weight, paper-weight, book) in your right hand.

○ Bending at the waist, place your left hand on a chair seat or other object of about the same height for balance.

○ With your right palm facing inward, lift your right hand up toward your right shoulder.

○ Lower your hand.

○ Repeat 12 to 20 times.

○ Repeat with your left arm.

With Exercise Tubing (or large rubber bands tied together)

○ Take the same position as described above. Do not hold a heavy object, though.

○ Instead, hold one end of the tubing (or rubber bands) in your right hand and hold down the other end with your left foot.

○ Pull your right hand up toward your right shoulder. Lower your hand.

○ Repeat 12 to 20 times.

○ Repeat with your left arm, holding down the tubing (or rubber bands) with your right foot.

Standing Push-up

○ Stand facing a wall (or a desk or copier), with your feet about 3 feet from the wall.

○ Place both palms on the wall at shoulder height and shoulder width apart. Keep your back straight.

○ Bending at the elbows, lean toward the wall. Hold for a second.

○ Push back from the wall until your arms are straight again.

○ Repeat 12 to 20 times.

Chair Dip

○ *Be sure your chair is completely secure.*

○ Sit on the front edge of the chair, with both feet on the floor. Your lower legs should be at right angles to your upper legs.

○ Put both hands on the front edge of the seat. Keep your arms straight.

○ Slowly lower your body toward the floor by bending your arms until your upper and lower arms are at right angles.

○ Slowly push up until your arms are straight again.

○ Repeat 8 to 12 times.

Leg Curl

○ Stand behind your chair and grab the chair back for balance.

○ Slowly lift your left foot toward your buttocks.

○ Lower your leg.

○ Repeat 12 to 20 times.

○ Repeat with your right foot.

Lunge

○ Put your hands on your hips (or hold onto a chair for balance if necessary).

○ Put your right foot forward about 3 feet.

○ Lower your left knee toward the floor without letting it touch the floor. Make sure your right knee does not go farther forward than your right toes.

○ Stand.

○ Repeat 8 to 12 times.

○ Repeat with left leg forward.

Half Squat

- ○ Stand with feet shoulder width apart.

- ○ Raise your arms in front of you and squat, bending your knees until your thighs are nearly parallel with the floor. (If necessary, hold on to a desk, chair, or other object for balance.) Be sure your knees do not extend farther forward than your toes.

- ○ Hold for 2 to 3 seconds, then stand straight.

- ○ Repeat 8 to 12 times.

Wall Sit

- ○ Stand with your back against a wall and your heels about 2 feet from the wall.

- ○ Bending your knees, slowly lower your upper body until you are in a seated position. Do not arch your back at any time.

- ○ Hold for 5 to 15 seconds.

- ○ Stand.

- ○ Repeat 3 to 5 times.

Calf Raise

- ○ Stand with your hands on your hips and your feet shoulder width apart.

- ○ Raise up on your toes, lifting your heels off the floor.

- ○ Lower your heels and repeat 12 to 20 times.

○ Variation: Stand on a book, curb, or stair step and let your heels hang off the edge. Raise and lower your heels as described above.

♡ *Stretching Activities*

Doing stretching activities is a great way to relieve tension and promote flexibility in your muscles and joints. When doing these stretching activities:

○ Do not bounce.

○ Use slow, controlled movements.

○ Stretch only until you feel a slight tension or pull. Do not try to force yourself beyond this point!

○ Hold each stretch 10 to 30 seconds.

Seated Activities

Neck Roll

○ Drop your chin to your chest and hold. Feel the stretch in the back of your neck.

○ Roll your head to the right and hold. Feel the stretch on the left side.

○ Roll your head to the front again and hold. Roll your head to the left and hold.

○ *Do not roll your head backward!* You could crush the vertebrae at the top of your spinal column.

Shoulder Roll

○ With your arms relaxed at your sides, rotate your right shoulder backward in a circular motion. Be sure to complete the circle while keeping your arm straight at your side.

○ Repeat 4 times.

○ Repeat with the left shoulder.

○ Roll both shoulders at the same time.

○ Repeat 3 to 5 times.

Shoulder Reach

○ Hold your arms straight in front of you with palms facing each other.

○ Interlace your fingers and rotate your palms so they face away from your body.

○ Extend your arms forward until you feel a stretch in your shoulders and arms.

○ Hold, then relax.

○ Repeat 10 times.

○ Raise your arms over your head with palms up.

○ Push your arms upward and slightly behind your head.

○ Hold, then relax.

○ Repeat 10 times.

Pretzel

○ Raise both arms above your head, fingers pointed to the ceiling.

○ Bend your right elbow, and put your right hand on the back of your neck.

○ Grab your right elbow with your left hand and gently pull your right elbow to the left. You should feel the stretch in the back of your upper right arm.

○ Hold, then relax.

○ Repeat 10 times.

○ Repeat 10 times with the left arm.

Wrist Roll

○ Make a loose fist with your right hand.

○ Holding your arm still, slowly rotate your hand in a circular motion at the wrist.

○ Repeat 10 times in each direction.

○ Repeat with your left hand.

Toe-Touch Stretch

○ Sitting toward the back of the chair, place your hands on your thighs.

○ With your left foot on the floor for balance, extend your right leg.

○ Bend forward slowly and reach for your right foot.

○ Hold.

○ Sit up slowly and put your right foot on the floor.

○ Repeat 4 times.

○ Repeat 4 times with your left leg.

Standing Activities

To get the full effect of these activities, take off your shoes.

Shoulder Stretch

○ Stand with your feet slightly apart.

○ Raise your right arm in front of you.

○ Bending at the elbow, bring your right arm across your chest at shoulder height until you feel a slight pull in your right shoulder.

○ Gently apply pressure with your left hand at your right elbow.

○ Hold, then relax.

○ Repeat 10 times.

○ Repeat on the left side 10 times.

Chest Stretch

○ Stand just outside an open doorway (the doorway should be behind you) and face outward.

○ Grab both sides of the door frame at chest height.

○ Take a step forward and let your arms straighten behind you. Keep your head up and lean forward until you feel a stretch in your chest muscles.

○ Hold, then relax.

○ Repeat 10 times.

Shoulder Pull

○ Stand just inside an open doorway (the doorway should be in front of you) and face outward.

○ Grab both sides of the door frame at chest height.

○ Lean back until you feel a stretch in your shoulder muscles.

○ Hold, then relax.

○ Repeat 5 to 10 times.

Side Bend

○ Stand with your feet 1 to 2 feet apart, with knees slightly bent.

○ Raise your right hand over your head and place your left hand on your left hip.

○ Lean to the left, bending slightly at the waist. Stop as soon as you feel a slight stretch in your right side.

○ Hold, slowly raise back up to vertical.

○ Repeat 5 to 10 times.

○ Repeat 5 to 10 times to the right side.

Back Arch

○ Stand with your feet shoulder width apart and knees slightly bent.

○ Place your hands on the front of your thighs and bend forward slightly at the waist, keeping your back flat.

○ Slowly inhale and arch your back.

○ Hold, then exhale.

○ Return to the flat back position.

○ Repeat 10 times.

Back Bend

○ Stand with your feet shoulder width apart and knees slightly bent.

○ Place your hands on your hips.

○ Lean backward slightly. *Be sure not to lean too far back!*

○ Hold, then relax.

○ Repeat 10 times.

Calf Stretch

○ Stand facing a wall, with your feet approximately 3 feet from the wall.

○ Place your hands on the wall at about shoulder height.

○ Keeping your feet flat on the floor, lean forward until you feel a slight stretch in your calves.

○ Hold, then relax.

○ Repeat 10 times.

Front Thigh Stretch

○ Stand facing a wall, with your feet approximately 3 feet from the wall.

○ Place your right hand on the wall at chest height.

○ Bend your left leg.

○ Use your left hand to grab the top of your left foot behind you.

○ Gently pull your heel toward your buttocks.

○ Hold, then relax.

○ Repeat 5 to 10 times.

○ Repeat 5 to 10 times on the other side.

Back Hamstring Stretch

○ Stand with your feet together and your hands on your hips.

○ Bending your right leg slightly, step forward with your left leg. Keep your left heel on the floor and your left toes pointed upward.

○ Put both hands on your right leg for balance, and gently sit back slightly, keeping your back straight.

○ Hold for 10 seconds.

○ Repeat with the other leg.

WALK YOUR WAY TO FITNESS

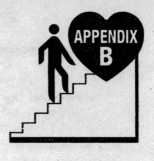

APPENDIX B

One good way to measure your fitness level is to try the 1-Mile Walking Test. First, though, you need to learn how to take your pulse (see the box below).

HOW TO TAKE YOUR PULSE

Where—Take your pulse on your neck, to the right or left of your Adam's apple, or on the inside of your wrist, on the thumb side.

How—Use the tips of your first two fingers (not your thumb) to press lightly over the blood vessels in your neck or on your wrist. Count your pulse for ten seconds and multiply by six. For example, if you counted 20 beats in ten seconds, your pulse would be 120 beats per minute.

When—If you can, keep walking while you take your pulse. You'll get a more accurate reading. Practice taking your pulse before you take the 1-Mile Walking Test.

The following checklist will help you get ready for the test:

_____ Set the course. Use a high school track (four laps = 1 mile) or a 1-mile track in a park, or drive and measure a 1-mile course that's safe and flat.

_____ Practice taking your pulse.

_____ Get a stopwatch or a watch with a second hand.

_____ Have a pencil and paper ready to write down your time and pulse.

_____ Be sure you have comfortable walking shoes.

A few factors can affect the accuracy of your test results:

○ If the weather is extremely hot, cold, humid, or windy, it will affect your performance. Go ahead and do your walk, then take the test a few days later when weather conditions improve.

○ Caffeine and alcohol can affect your heart rate, and a heavy meal can make you uncomfortable when you exercise. Avoid all of them for three to four hours before walking.

○ Any medication that raises or lowers your heart rate will make the test inaccurate.

♡ Taking the Test

Warm up for a few minutes with both easy walking and stretching exercises. Begin your test by walking quickly at a steady pace to get your pulse to 110 beats per minute. Walk at a "conversation pace" (you should be able to talk while walking). If you cannot talk while walking, slow down until you can.

After five minutes, take your pulse. It should still be at 110 beats per minute or higher. As you cross the 1-mile mark, check the time it took you to walk in both minutes and seconds. Keep walking but at a slower pace to cool down. Take your pulse again when you cross the mark or after cooling down.

Assume that you're a forty-year-old woman who walked the mile in 19:00 minutes. When you checked your pulse at the end of the test, it was 140 beats per minute. Your record would look like this:

The 1-Mile Walking Test Data Record

Interval	Date	Time	Pulse	Fitness Level Category	Other
Baseline	3/2	19:00	140	low*	
One Month					
Two Months					
Three Months					

*See pages 157–159 for how to figure out your fitness level category.

Record your scores and track your progress in Appendix C.

After you complete the 1-Mile Walking Test, you'll have a good idea of your current fitness level. Repeat the test after four to six weeks of fitting in fitness. If you walk the mile faster and/or your pulse is slower, give yourself a pat on the back—you've improved your fitness level.

♡ Scoring the 1 – Mile Walking Test

 Find your age group in the table on the facing page.

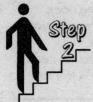 Round off your heart rate to the nearest 10 beats (for example, for 133 beats per minute, use 130 beats per minute).

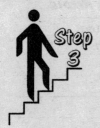 Find your fitness level by referring to the appropriate A and B columns.

If your time for walking the mile was the same as for column A or if it took you longer, you're in the **low fitness** category.

If you walked the mile between the times listed in columns A and B, you're in the **moderate fitness** category.

If your walking time matches or is less than the time in column B, you're in the **high fitness** category.

		Men		Women	
Age	Heart Rate	A	B	A	B
20–29	110	19:36	17:06	20:57	19:08
	120	19:10	16:36	20:27	18:38
	130	18:35	16:06	20:00	18:12
	140	18:06	15:36	19:30	17:42
	150	17:36	15:10	19:00	17:12
	160	17:09	14:42	18:30	16:42
	170	16:39	14:12	18:00	16:12
30–39	110	18:21	15:54	19:46	17:52
	120	17:52	15:24	19:18	17:24
	130	17:22	14:54	18:48	16:54
	140	16:54	14:30	18:18	16:24
	150	16:26	14:00	17:48	15:54
	160	15:58	13:30	17:18	15:24
	170	15:28	13:01	16:54	14:55
40–49	110	18:05	15:38	19:15	17:20
	120	17:36	15:09	18:45	16:50
	130	17:07	14:41	18:18	16:24
	140	16:38	14:12	17:48	15:54
	150	16:09	13:42	17:18	15:24
	160	15:42	13:15	16:48	14:54
	170	15:12	12:45	16:18	14:25
50–59	110	17:49	15:22	18:40	17:04
	120	17:20	14:53	18:12	16:36
	130	16:51	14:24	17:42	16:06
	140	16:22	13:51	17:18	15:36
	150	15:53	13:26	16:48	15:06
	160	15:26	12:59	16:18	14:36
	170	14:56	12:30	15:48	14:06

(table continued)

		Men		Women	
Age	**Heart Rate**	**A**	**B**	**A**	**B**
60+	110	17:55	15:33	18:00	16:36
	120	17:24	15:04	17:30	16:06
	130	16:57	14:36	17:01	15:37
	140	16:28	14:07	16:31	15:09
	150	15:59	13:39	16:02	14:39
	160	15:30	13:10	15:32	14:12
	170	15:04	12:42	15:04	13:42

The 1-Mile Walking Test is adapted with permission from fitness standards developed by the Cooper Institute for Aerobics Research, Dallas, Texas. All rights reserved. The test is based on maximal oxygen uptake estimates from studies done by Dr. James M. Rippe and colleagues. *Journal of the American Medical Association, 259:* 2720–2724, 1988.

1-Mile Walking Test Data Record

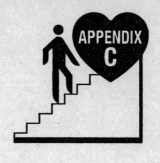

Interval	Date	Time	Pulse	Fitness Category	Other
Baseline					
One Month					
Two Months					
Three Months					
Four Months					
Five Months					
Six Months					
Seven Months					
Eight Months					
Nine Months					
Ten Months					
Eleven Months					
One Year					

WEEKLY PHYSICAL ACTIVITY DIARY

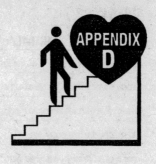

Here are some sample entries for a weekly physical activity diary. Starting on page 166, you'll find a clean diary for recording your accomplishments.

WEEKLY GOAL(S) <u>ride stationary bike while on the</u>

<u>telephone, do 15 min. of activity per day</u>

_____

SUNDAY <u>2/9</u>

ACTIVITY	MINUTES
walked around soccer field during son's game	18
rode stationary bike while on telephone	10
TOTAL MINUTES	28

Comments:_____

MONDAY 2 /10

ACTIVITY	MINUTES
parked at far end of parking lot at work and walked	3
took stairs to/from meeting on third floor	2
walked around building during lunch	7
stretched while copying	2
rode stationary bike while watching TV	10
TOTAL MINUTES	24

Comments: felt energized after lunch

SATURDAY 2 / 15

ACTIVITY	MINUTES
parked at grocery store, walked to bank and cleaners, walked through grocery store, carried bags to car	32
walked around restaurant parking lot while waiting to be seated	10
TOTAL MINUTES	42

Comments: enjoyed dinner after walking

<u>WEEKLY SUMMARY</u>

GOAL(S) ATTAINED

☑ YES   ☐ SOME/ALMOST   ☐ NO

ACTIVITIES INCLUDED

☑ CARDIOVASCULAR

☑ STRENGTH

☑ FLEXIBILITY/STRETCHING

NEW ACTIVITY(IES) INCLUDED   walking in parking lot at

restaurant

_____

_____

_____

_____

_____

_____

_____

_____

REWARD bought water bottle for work

_____

_____

SUNDAY____/____

ACTIVITY	MINUTES
TOTAL MINUTES	

Comments:_____

MONDAY____/____

ACTIVITY	MINUTES
TOTAL MINUTES	

Comments:_____

TUESDAY___/___

ACTIVITY	MINUTES
TOTAL MINUTES	

Comments:_____

WEDNESDAY___/___

ACTIVITY	MINUTES
TOTAL MINUTES	

Comments:_____

THURSDAY___/___

ACTIVITY	MINUTES
TOTAL MINUTES	

Comments:_____

FRIDAY___/___

ACTIVITY	MINUTES
TOTAL MINUTES	

Comments:_____

SATURDAY___/___

ACTIVITY	MINUTES
TOTAL MINUTES	

Comments:_____

WEEKLY SUMMARY

GOAL(S) ATTAINED

☐ YES ☐ SOME/ALMOST ☐ NO

ACTIVITIES INCLUDED

☐ CARDIOVASCULAR

☐ STRENGTH

☐ FLEXIBILITY/STRETCHING

NEW ACTIVITY(IES) INCLUDED _____

_____

_____

_____

_____

_____

_____

_____

_____

_____

REWARD _____

_____

_____

WHERE TO REACH US

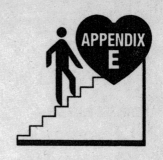

For information about the
American Heart Association,
call 1-800-AHA-USA1
(1-800-242-8721) or
contact us online at
http://www.amhrt.org.